AF782344

Understanding Postpartum Adjustment

A Guide to Managing and Living with the Challenges of the Fourth Trimester

Kaida Mabry

Xspurts.com

Created by Xspurts.com

A New Zealand Designed Product

Other Versions Available

Why limit yourself to just one format?

This book is now available in physical, digital, and audiobook options.

Choose the way you love to read and dive into the story today. You won't regret it!

Digital ISBN: 9781776848157
Physical ISBN: 9781776847068
Audio ISBN:

To obtain a different format of this book at a discounted price, please get in touch with us at:

http://isbn.xspurts.com/

Contents

Have Questions / Comments?

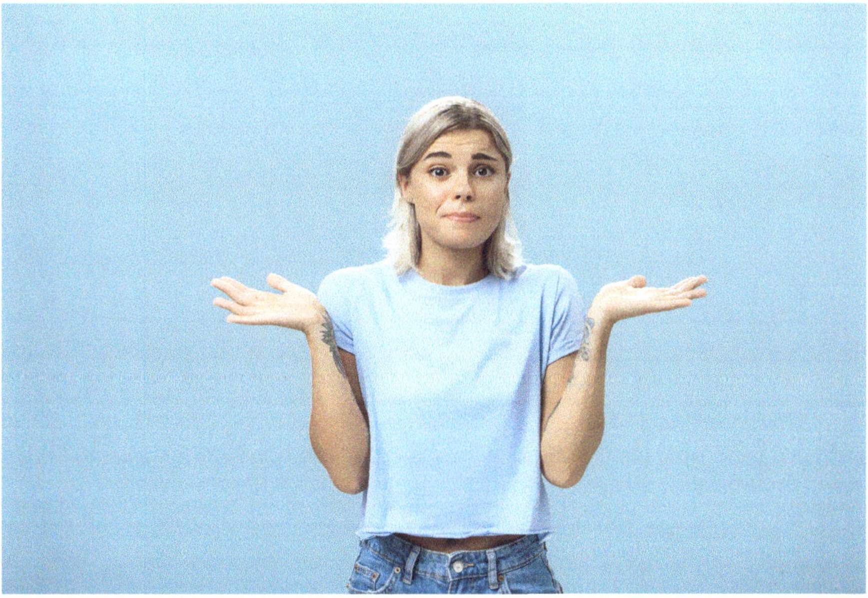

This book was designed to cover as much information as possible, but I know I have probably missed something, or some new amazing discovery has just come out.

If you notice something missing or have a question that I failed to answer, please get in touch and let me know. If I can, I will email you an answer and also update the book so others can also benefit from it.

Thanks For Being Awesome :)

Submit Your Questions / Comments At:

https://questions.xspurts.com

Get Free Stuff

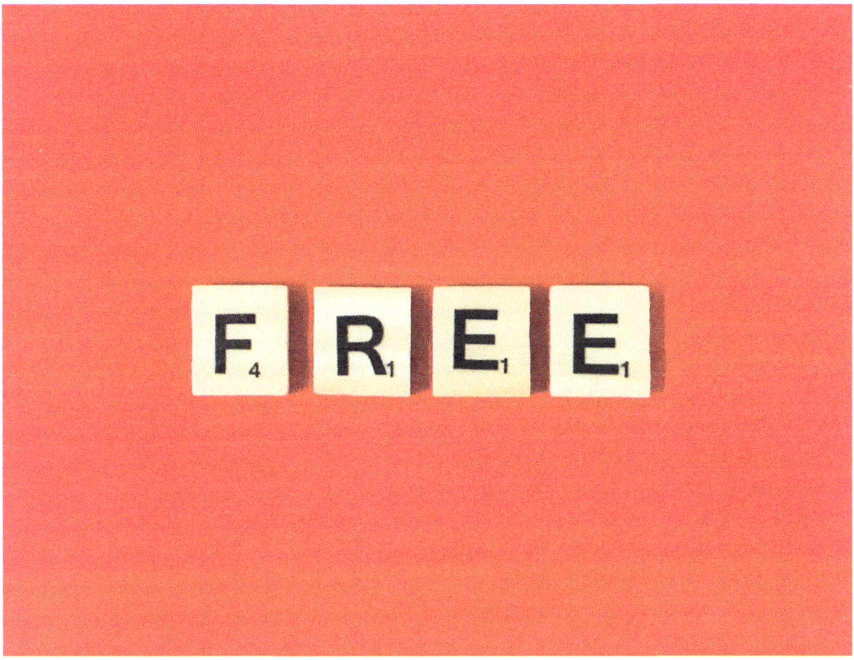

We love writing and have produced a huge number of books.

For being one of our amazing readers, we would love to offer you more books we have created, 100% free.

To claim this limited time special offer, simply go to the site below and enter your name and email address.

You will then receive loads (as we love our readers so much :) of our great books, content and audio direct to your email account, 100% free!

Get Loads of FREE Stuff at:

https://free.xspurts.com

Chapter One

Understanding Postpartum Period

The postpartum period, often referred to as the "fourth trimester," is a crucial time of adjustment and healing for new mothers. It is a phase that encompasses physical, emotional, and hormonal changes as a woman transitions from pregnancy to motherhood. Understanding the postpartum period is essential not only for the well, being of new mothers but also for their successful recovery and the establishment of a strong bond with their newborns. Below we will delve into the various aspects of the postpartum period, shedding light on its significance, challenges, and strategies for postpartum recovery.

Physical Recovery:

a. Involution of the Uterus: After giving birth, the uterus undergoes a process known as involution, where it gradually returns to its pre, pregnancy size. This process involves the shedding of the uterine lining and the contraction of uterine muscles. Understanding this natural process helps new mothers appreciate their bodies' ability to heal and recover.

b. Postpartum Bleeding: Following childbirth, new mothers experience postpartum bleeding, known as lochia. Lochia consists of blood, mucus, and tissue that was present in the uterus during pregnancy. This discharge can last for several weeks and gradually transitions from bright red to pink and then to a yellowish, white color. Awareness of this normal postpartum occurrence helps alleviate concerns and promotes a sense of reassurance.

c. Perineal Healing: If a woman has experienced perineal tearing or an episiotomy during childbirth, the perineum requires time to heal. This area may be sore, swollen, and tender. Understanding the importance of proper perineal care, including keeping the area clean and using pain relief measures, aids in the healing process.

Emotional Adjustments:

a. Postpartum Blues: Many new mothers experience the "baby blues," a temporary emotional state characterized by mood swings, tearfulness, and feelings of vulnerability. These feelings usually subside within a few weeks as hormone levels stabilize. Recognizing and acknowledging the baby blues as a normal part of the postpartum period helps new mothers navigate this emotional transition.

b. Postpartum Depression: Postpartum depression is a more severe and long, lasting condition that affects some new mothers. It involves persistent feelings of sadness, fatigue, loss of interest, and difficulty bonding with the baby. Recognizing the symptoms of postpartum depression and seeking professional help is crucial to ensure appropriate support and treatment.

c. Hormonal Changes: Hormonal fluctuations during the postpartum period, particularly a decrease in estrogen and progesterone levels, can impact mood and emotions. Understanding these hormonal changes helps new mothers contextualize their emotional experiences and seek appropriate support when needed.

Breastfeeding and Infant Care:

a. Breastfeeding Challenges: The postpartum period is a critical time for establishing breastfeeding. New mothers may encounter challenges such as latching difficulties, engorgement, or nipple soreness. Educating oneself about proper breastfeeding techniques, seeking support from lactation consultants, and joining breastfeeding support groups can greatly assist in overcoming these challenges.

b. Newborn Care: Caring for a newborn can be overwhelming, particularly for first, time mothers. Understanding the basics of infant care, including feeding schedules, diaper changes, and soothing techniques, provides new mothers with the confidence and knowledge needed to meet their baby's needs.

c. Sleep Deprivation: Sleep disruptions are a common aspect of the postpartum period due to the demands of caring for a newborn. Understanding strategies for managing sleep deprivation, such as prioritizing rest, napping when the baby sleeps, and seeking help from partners or support systems, can mitigate the effects of sleep deprivation on new mothers' well, being.

Physical Changes After Birth

The journey of pregnancy and childbirth is a remarkable experience that brings about significant physical changes to a woman's body. Following the birth of a baby, new mothers embark on a transformative postpartum period characterized by further physical adjustments and the process of recovery. Understanding these physical changes is crucial for postpartum recovery, self, care, and adjusting to the new demands of motherhood. Below we will explore the fascinating physical changes that occur after birth and discuss strategies for navigating the postpartum recovery journey.

Uterine Changes:

a. Uterine Involution: After childbirth, the uterus begins a process called involution, where it gradually contracts to its pre, pregnancy size. This process is essential for the body to return to its normal state. Understanding the importance of uterine involution helps new mothers appreciate their bodies' ability to heal and recover.

b. Lochia Discharge: Following delivery, new mothers experience lochia, which is a discharge consisting of blood, tissue, and mucus from the site where the placenta was attached. The color and amount of lochia change over time, transitioning from bright red to pinkish, brown and eventually to a yellowish, white discharge. Awareness of this normal postpartum occurrence aids in identifying any abnormal changes and promotes proper hygiene during the recovery period.

Breast Changes:

a. Engorgement: In the early postpartum days, breast engorgement is a common occurrence as the breasts fill with milk. This can result in feelings of fullness, tenderness, and even pain. Understanding strategies for managing engorgement, such as breastfeeding frequently, using warm compresses, and expressing milk, helps alleviate discomfort and prevent complications like mastitis.

b. Milk Production: The body undergoes significant changes to support milk production and breastfeeding. The hormone prolactin stimulates milk production, while oxytocin triggers the let, down reflex, allowing milk to flow. Recognizing the body's natural mechanisms for milk production and understanding the importance of establishing a breastfeeding routine promotes successful breastfeeding and fosters bonding with the baby.

Hormonal Adjustments:

a. Estrogen and Progesterone: The hormonal balance in a woman's body undergoes a dramatic shift after birth. Estrogen and progesterone levels, which were significantly elevated during pregnancy, decrease rapidly. These hormonal adjustments can affect mood, energy levels, and even hair growth. Recognizing the influence of hormones on the postpartum experience helps new mothers navigate the emotional and physical changes they may encounter.

b. Prolactin and Oxytocin: Hormones such as prolactin and oxytocin play crucial roles in breastfeeding and bonding with the baby. Prolactin stimulates milk production, while oxytocin promotes the release of milk and facilitates the mother, infant bond. Understanding the function of these hormones enhances new mothers' confidence in their ability to breastfeed and fosters a deeper connection with their baby.

Abdominal and Pelvic Changes:

a. Abdominal Muscle Separation: During pregnancy, the abdominal muscles stretch and separate to accommodate the growing baby. This condition, known as diastasis recti, may persist after childbirth, resulting in a gap between the abdominal muscles. Engaging in specific exercises, such as core strengthening and pelvic floor exercises, under the guidance of a healthcare professional can assist in restoring abdominal muscle tone and function.

b. Pelvic Floor Recovery: The pelvic floor muscles, which support the pelvic organs, undergo significant strain during pregnancy and childbirth. This can lead to issues like urinary incontinence or pelvic organ prolapse. Understanding the importance of pelvic floor exercises, seeking guidance from a healthcare provider, and incorporating appropriate exercises into daily routines.

Emotional Changes After Birth

The postpartum period is a time of immense joy, love, and excitement as new parents welcome their precious bundle of joy. However, it is also a phase characterized by a range of emotional changes that can sometimes catch new mothers off guard. Understanding these emotional changes is essential for postpartum recovery, bonding with the baby, and seeking appropriate support. Below we will explore the fascinating emotional changes that occur after birth and discuss strategies for navigating the emotional rollercoaster of the postpartum period.

Baby Blues:

a. Baby blues are common and temporary mood swings that affect many new mothers. These feelings of sadness, irritability, and vulnerability usually emerge within the first week after giving birth and may last up to two weeks. Understanding that baby blues are a normal response to the hormonal shifts and adjustments of becoming a mother can provide reassurance during this emotional phase.

b. Self, care, emotional support from loved ones, and open communication about feelings can help new mothers navigate the baby blues. Recognizing the temporary nature of these emotions and seeking support can significantly alleviate distress during this period.

Postpartum Depression:

a. Postpartum depression (PPD) is a more severe and persistent form of emotional distress that affects some new mothers. It is characterized by intense feelings of sadness, hopelessness, fatigue, and a loss of interest in activities. PPD can significantly impact a mother's well, being and ability to care for herself and her baby.

b. Recognizing the signs of PPD, including persistent symptoms lasting longer than two weeks, is crucial for early intervention and treatment. Seeking professional help from healthcare providers, therapists, or support groups can provide the necessary support and treatment options for managing PPD.

Anxiety and Worry:

a. It is common for new mothers to experience anxiety and worry about their baby's health, well, being, and their own abilities as a parent. The responsibility of caring for a newborn, combined with hormonal fluctuations and sleep deprivation, can contribute to heightened levels of anxiety.

b. Developing coping strategies, such as deep breathing exercises, mindfulness practices, and seeking reassurance from healthcare providers, can help manage anxiety and promote a sense of calm. Engaging in self, care activities and ensuring adequate rest can also alleviate stress and anxiety.

Identity and Self, esteem:

a. The transition to motherhood can bring about a significant shift in a woman's identity and self, esteem. Balancing the demands of motherhood with personal goals, career aspirations, and self, care can sometimes lead to a sense of loss or identity confusion.

b. It is important for new mothers to engage in self, reflection and self, compassion, acknowledging that their identity has expanded rather than diminished. Setting realistic expectations, celebrating personal achievements, and seeking support from loved ones can foster a positive sense of self during the postpartum period.

Relationship Changes:

a. The arrival of a baby can impact relationships, including those with partners, family members, and friends. Adjusting to the new dynamics of parenthood can lead to changes in communication, division of responsibilities, and intimacy.

b. Open and honest communication with partners and loved ones is key to navigating relationship changes. Setting aside dedicated time for connection, seeking support from friends or support groups, and seeking couples counseling if needed can help strengthen relationships during this transition.

Seeking Support:

a. Recognizing the importance of seeking emotional support is vital during the postpartum period. Connecting with other new mothers through support groups, online communities, or social networks can provide validation, encouragement, and a sense of camaraderie.

b. Seeking support from healthcare professionals, therapists, or counselors can offer guidance and coping strategies for managing emotional changes.

Chapter Two

The Importance of Self, Care

The postpartum period is a time of profound change and adjustment for new mothers. As they dedicate themselves to the care and well, being of their newborns, it is crucial not to overlook their own physical, emotional, and mental health. Self, care plays a vital role in postpartum recovery, allowing new mothers to replenish their energy, foster emotional well, being, and navigate the challenges of motherhood with resilience. Below we will explore the importance of self, care during the postpartum period and discuss practical strategies for incorporating self, care into the daily lives of new mothers.

Physical Self, Care:

a. Rest and Sleep: Adequate rest and sleep are essential for postpartum recovery. New mothers often experience sleep deprivation due to frequent nighttime feedings and caring for their newborns. Prioritizing rest, taking naps when the baby sleeps, and enlisting the support of partners or loved ones can help new mothers replenish their energy levels.

b. Nutrition and Hydration: Nourishing the body with nutritious food and staying hydrated are vital for postpartum recovery. New mothers should focus on consuming a well, balanced diet rich in fruits, vegetables, lean proteins, and whole grains. Drinking plenty of water and limiting caffeine intake are also important for overall well, being.

c. Gentle Exercise: Engaging in gentle exercise, with the approval of healthcare providers, can have numerous benefits for postpartum recovery. Activities like walking, yoga, or postnatal exercises can help restore muscle tone, improve mood, and increase energy levels. New mothers should start slowly and gradually increase the intensity of their exercise routine.

Emotional and Mental Self, Care:

a. Prioritizing Emotional Well, being: It is essential for new mothers to prioritize their emotional well, being. Engaging in activities that bring joy, practicing mindfulness or meditation, and seeking support from loved ones or support groups can promote emotional well, being. Journaling or talking to a therapist can also provide a safe space to express emotions and navigate the challenges of motherhood.

b. Setting Boundaries: New mothers often face numerous demands on their time and energy. Setting boundaries and learning to say "no" to non, essential commitments can help protect their emotional well, being. Prioritizing self, care activities and delegating tasks to partners or loved ones can create space for new mothers to recharge and focus on their own needs.

c. Seeking Support: It is important for new mothers to seek support from healthcare professionals, therapists, or counselors if they are experiencing difficulties or struggling with their mental health. Recognizing the signs of postpartum depression or anxiety and reaching out for professional help can make a significant difference in the recovery process.

Social and Relationship Self, Care:

a. Nurturing Relationships: Maintaining healthy relationships with partners, family members, and friends is crucial during the postpartum period. Spending quality time with loved ones, engaging in activities that foster connection, and seeking emotional support can help new mothers feel supported and reduce feelings of isolation.

b. Connecting with Other Mothers: Building a community of other new mothers can provide a valuable support system. Joining mother's groups, attending parenting classes, or participating in online forums can create opportunities for sharing experiences, receiving advice, and forming lasting friendships.

c. Me, Time: Carving out time for oneself is a vital aspect of self, care. Whether it's taking a relaxing bath, reading a book, pursuing a hobby, or simply enjoying a cup of tea, me, time allows new mothers to recharge and reconnect with themselves. Partners or family members can help by taking on caregiving responsibilities, allowing new mothers to have uninterrupted time for self, care activities.

Rest and Sleep

Revitalizing the Body and Mind: Exploring the Significance of Rest and Sleep in Postpartum Recovery

The postpartum period is a time of immense joy, wonder, and adjustment for new mothers. Amidst the joy of welcoming a newborn, it is crucial for mothers to prioritize their own physical and mental well, being. Rest and sleep play a pivotal role in postpartum recovery, aiding in the healing process, enhancing emotional resilience, and promoting overall health. Below we will delve into the importance of rest and sleep during the postpartum period and discuss strategies to optimize these essential elements of self, care.

Physical Recovery:

a. Healing and Repair: Pregnancy and childbirth exert tremendous physical demands on a woman's body. Rest and sleep provide an opportunity for the body to heal and repair itself. Adequate rest allows the body to recover from the strain of labor, heal incisions or tears, and restore energy levels. It is during rest that the body produces growth hormones and engages in cellular regeneration, supporting the body's recovery process.

b. Hormonal Balance: Sleep is intricately linked to hormonal balance. The production of growth hormone, which aids in tissue repair, peaks during deep sleep. Restful sleep also supports the regulation of other hormones, such as cortisol and melatonin, which play a role in stress management and maintaining the body's natural rhythm. Achieving a balance in hormonal levels through adequate sleep contributes to the overall well, being of new mothers.

Emotional Well, being:

a. Hormonal Regulation: The postpartum period is characterized by significant hormonal fluctuations, including a decline in estrogen and progesterone levels. Sleep helps regulate these hormones, influencing mood and emotional stability. Sufficient sleep enhances serotonin production, promoting feelings of well, being, and reducing the risk of mood disorders such as postpartum depression.

b. Stress Reduction: Sleep plays a vital role in managing stress. The demands of caring for a newborn, coupled with sleep deprivation, can lead to heightened stress levels. Rest and sleep provide an opportunity for the body and mind to relax, reducing cortisol levels and alleviating stress. Prioritizing sleep can help new mothers cope with the emotional challenges and responsibilities of motherhood.

Cognitive Function:

a. Memory Consolidation: Restful sleep is essential for memory consolidation and cognitive function. During sleep, the brain processes and stores information gathered during wakefulness, aiding in learning and memory formation. Adequate sleep enhances cognitive abilities such as problem, solving, decision, making, and attention span, helping new mothers navigate the daily challenges of caring for their newborns.

b. Mental Clarity: Sleep deprivation can lead to cognitive impairments, including difficulty with concentration, reduced creativity, and impaired judgment. Sufficient rest allows the brain to recharge, enhancing mental clarity, and promoting optimal cognitive performance. By prioritizing sleep, new mothers can approach their responsibilities with clarity and focus.

Tips for Rest and Sleep Optimization:

a. Establish a Routine: Creating a consistent sleep routine helps signal to the body that it is time to rest. Establishing a regular bedtime and waking up time, even if sleep interruptions are frequent, can help regulate the body's internal clock and promote better sleep patterns over time.

b. Create a Restful Environment: Designing a soothing and comfortable sleep environment is crucial for quality rest. Dim the lights, reduce noise, and create a relaxing atmosphere conducive to sleep. Investing in a supportive mattress, breathable bedding, and appropriate sleepwear can enhance comfort and promote better sleep quality.

c. Share Responsibilities: Enlist the support of partners, family members, or friends to share caregiving responsibilities. This allows new mothers to take breaks and rest when needed. Communicate your needs and establish a support system that promotes rest and sleep.

Nutrition for Healing

The postpartum period is a time of immense physical and emotional changes for new mothers. As the body recovers from pregnancy and childbirth, proper nutrition plays a crucial role in supporting the healing process and restoring vitality. A well, balanced diet rich in essential nutrients not only promotes postpartum recovery but also provides the energy and nourishment needed to meet the demands of caring for a newborn. Below we will explore the significance of nutrition for healing during the postpartum period and provide practical tips for nourishing the body and promoting overall well, being.

Meeting Increased Nutritional Needs:

a. Adequate Caloric Intake: After giving birth, a woman's caloric needs are higher than during pregnancy. Lactation, physical recovery, and increased energy expenditure from caring for a newborn require additional calories. It is important to consume nutrient, dense foods to meet these increased energy requirements.

b. Macronutrients: A balanced postpartum diet should include an appropriate balance of macronutrients – carbohydrates, proteins, and fats. Carbohydrates provide energy, while proteins aid in tissue repair and hormone production. Healthy fats support brain function and hormone regulation. Choosing whole grains, lean proteins, and healthy fats ensures a well, rounded diet.

Essential Nutrients for Healing:

a. Iron: Iron is crucial for postpartum recovery, especially if there was significant blood loss during childbirth. Iron, rich foods, such as lean meats, poultry, fish, legumes, and dark leafy greens, should be included in the diet to replenish iron stores and prevent anemia.

b. Calcium and Vitamin D: Adequate calcium and vitamin D intake are important for bone health, particularly if breastfeeding. Dairy products, fortified plant, based milk, leafy greens, and seafood are excellent sources of calcium. Exposure to sunlight and fortified foods help fulfill the body's vitamin D requirements.

c. Omega, 3 Fatty Acids: Omega, 3 fatty acids have anti, inflammatory properties and promote brain health. Fatty fish, flaxseeds, chia seeds, and walnuts are rich sources of omega, 3s. Including these foods in the diet can support postpartum healing and potentially alleviate postpartum depression symptoms.

d. Fiber: Adequate fiber intake helps prevent constipation, a common issue during the postpartum period. Whole grains, fruits, vegetables, legumes, and nuts are high in fiber and support digestive health.

Hydration:

a. Drinking plenty of water is essential for postpartum recovery. Proper hydration aids in tissue repair, digestion, and milk production for breastfeeding mothers. It is recommended to consume at least eight glasses (64 ounces) of water per day, adjusting the intake as needed based on individual circumstances.

b. Herbal teas and fruit, infused water can add variety to hydration routines. Avoiding excessive caffeine and sugary beverages is important for overall hydration and well, being.

Meal Planning and Preparation:

a. Meal planning and preparation can greatly assist new mothers in maintaining a nutritious diet. Plan meals and snacks ahead of time to ensure a variety of nutrient, rich options are available.

b. Stocking the pantry and refrigerator with healthy staples such as whole grains, lean proteins, fruits, vegetables, and healthy snacks makes it easier to choose nourishing options.

c. Preparing meals in advance or accepting help from loved ones can alleviate the stress of cooking while adjusting to the demands of motherhood.

Incorporating Superfoods:

a. Superfoods are nutrient, dense foods that offer various health benefits. Incorporating these foods into the postpartum diet can enhance recovery and provide essential nutrients.

b. Examples of superfoods include berries, spinach, kale, avocados.

Chapter Three

Postpartum Body Changes

The journey of motherhood is a transformative and awe, inspiring experience. Alongside the joy and fulfillment that comes with welcoming a newborn, the postpartum period brings about significant changes in a woman's body. These changes are natural and necessary for the recovery and adaptation to the new role of motherhood. Understanding the postpartum body changes is crucial for promoting self, acceptance, facilitating recovery, and embracing the incredible strength and resilience of the female body. Below we will explore the fascinating postpartum body changes, shedding light on their purpose and providing insights into postpartum recovery.

Uterine Changes:

During pregnancy, the uterus expands to accommodate the growing baby. After childbirth, the uterus undergoes involution, gradually returning to its pre, pregnancy size. This process is facilitated by contractions, which help expel the placenta and compress the blood vessels to reduce bleeding. It typically takes about six weeks for the uterus to shrink back to its pre, pregnancy size.

Lochia:

Lochia refers to the vaginal discharge that occurs after childbirth. It consists of blood, tissue, and mucus from the healing uterus. Initially, the discharge is bright red and heavy, resembling a heavy menstrual period.

Over time, it transitions to a pinkish or brownish color and eventually becomes white or yellowish. Lochia typically lasts for four to six weeks and gradually decreases in volume as the body heals.

Breast Changes:

a. Engorgement: In the early postpartum period, the breasts may become engorged as they transition from producing colostrum to mature milk. This can result in feelings of fullness, tenderness, and swelling. Regular breastfeeding or pumping can help relieve engorgement.

b. Milk Production: As a response to the baby's demand for milk, the body begins producing mature milk within a few days after delivery. This process is facilitated by hormonal signals triggered by breastfeeding or pumping. The breasts may feel heavier, and milk may leak between feedings. Establishing a breastfeeding routine helps regulate milk production and supply.

Hormonal Changes:

a. Estrogen and Progesterone: The levels of estrogen and progesterone drop significantly after childbirth. These hormonal changes can contribute to mood swings, emotional changes, and potentially postpartum depression. It is important to seek support and communicate feelings with healthcare providers, as they can provide guidance and resources for managing these changes.

b. Prolactin: Prolactin is the hormone responsible for milk production. Its levels increase to stimulate breast milk production in response to breastfeeding or pumping. Prolactin also has a calming effect and promotes bonding between mother and baby.

Abdominal Changes:

a. Diastasis Recti: Diastasis recti refers to the separation of the abdominal muscles that occurs during pregnancy. After childbirth, these muscles gradually come back together. However, in some cases, the separation may persist, leading to a bulging or protruding abdomen. Engaging in appropriate exercises and seeking guidance from healthcare professionals can aid in the healing of diastasis recti.

b. Stretch Marks: Stretch marks are a common occurrence during pregnancy, resulting from the stretching of the skin as the baby grows. These marks may fade over time but often remain as a reminder of the miraculous journey of motherhood.

Pelvic Floor Changes:

a. Weakness and Pelvic Organ Prolapse: Pregnancy and childbirth can weaken the pelvic floor muscles. This can lead to symptoms such as urinary incontinence, pelvic pressure, or prolapse. Engaging in pelvic floor exercises, such as Kegels, and seek guidance from healthcare providers or pelvic floor therapists.

Skin and Hair Changes

The journey of motherhood is filled with incredible moments and precious memories. Alongside the joy and fulfillment, the postpartum period brings about notable changes in a woman's body, including the skin and hair. These changes are a natural part of the postpartum recovery process and can vary from woman to woman. Understanding and embracing these transformations can help new mothers navigate their postpartum journey with confidence and self, acceptance. Below we will explore the fascinating skin and hair changes that occur during the postpartum period, shedding light on their causes and providing insights into postpartum recovery.

Skin Changes:

a. Stretch Marks: One of the most common skin changes during pregnancy is the development of stretch marks. These reddish or purplish lines appear on the abdomen, breasts, hips, and thighs due to the stretching of the skin as the baby grows. Although they may fade over time, stretch marks are a natural part of the postpartum body and serve as a reminder of the incredible journey of motherhood.

b. Pigmentation Changes: Hormonal fluctuations during pregnancy can lead to changes in skin pigmentation. Many women experience darkening of the skin, particularly around the areolas, armpits, and inner thighs. This condition, known as hyperpigmentation, is typically temporary and may fade in the months following childbirth.

c. Acne and Oiliness: Hormonal changes during pregnancy and the postpartum period can contribute to changes in skin oil production. Some women may experience increased acne or oiliness, while others may notice improvements in their skin condition. Establishing a consistent skincare routine and consulting with a dermatologist can help manage these changes.

d. Dryness and Sensitivity: Hormonal fluctuations can also result in dry and sensitive skin. It is important to moisturize regularly and use gentle, hypoallergenic skincare products to maintain the skin's moisture balance. Drinking plenty of water and incorporating foods rich in antioxidants can also support skin health.

Hair Changes:

a. Hair Loss: Many women experience postpartum hair loss, known as telogen effluvium, in the months following childbirth. During pregnancy, elevated estrogen levels prolong the hair growth phase, resulting in thick, lustrous hair. However, after childbirth, hormonal changes cause a significant number of hairs to enter the resting phase, leading to hair shedding. This hair loss is temporary and typically resolves within a few months.

b. Changes in Hair Texture: Hormonal fluctuations can also impact hair texture. Some women may notice changes in hair thickness, curl pattern, or oiliness. These changes are temporary and generally revert to normal as hormone levels stabilize.

c. Hair Growth: After the postpartum hair loss phase, many women experience regrowth of new hair. It is important to nourish the hair with a balanced diet, rich in vitamins and minerals, to support healthy hair growth. Being gentle with the hair and avoiding excessive heat styling can also promote hair health.

Self, Care Tips for Skin and Hair:

a. Skincare Routine: Establishing a consistent skincare routine can help maintain skin health during the postpartum period. Cleanse the skin with gentle, pH, balanced cleansers, moisturize daily, and use sunscreen to protect the skin from UV damage. If specific skin concerns arise, consulting with a dermatologist can provide personalized guidance.

b. Healthy Nutrition: A balanced diet is crucial for skin and hair health. Consuming a variety of nutrient, rich foods, including fruits, vegetables, whole grains, lean proteins, and healthy fats, provides the body with essential vitamins and minerals necessary for optimal skin and hair function.

c. Hydration: Drinking plenty of water is essential for overall health.

Weight Management

Navigating Weight Management: Balancing Health and Well, being in Postpartum Recovery

The postpartum period is a time of profound physical and emotional changes for new mothers. As the body adjusts to its pre, pregnancy state, weight management becomes a topic of concern for many women. It is important to approach weight management during postpartum recovery with a focus on overall health, well, being, and self, compassion. Below we will explore the complexities of weight management in the postpartum period, providing factual information, practical tips, and emphasizing the importance of a balanced approach to support a healthy and positive postpartum recovery.

Understanding Weight Fluctuations:

a. Pregnancy, Related Weight Loss: Immediately after childbirth, women may experience significant weight loss due to the elimination of the baby, amniotic fluid, and placenta. Additionally, the body sheds excess fluid accumulated during pregnancy. This initial weight loss can range from 10 to 15 pounds or more.

b. Breastfeeding and Caloric Expenditure: Breastfeeding can aid in postpartum weight loss as it burns additional calories. However, the impact on weight loss varies from person to person, and it is important to prioritize a balanced diet rather than focusing solely on weight reduction.

c. Retaining Weight for Lactation: The body naturally retains some weight during breastfeeding to support milk production. This is a normal and essential part of the lactation process.

Nourishing the Body:

a. Balanced Diet: Adopting a balanced and nutrient, rich diet is crucial for postpartum recovery and overall well, being. Focus on consuming a variety of fruits, vegetables, whole grains, lean proteins, and healthy fats. Avoid restrictive diets, as they may negatively impact milk production and overall energy levels.

b. Portion Control: Paying attention to portion sizes can help regulate caloric intake without compromising nutrition. Listening to hunger and fullness cues and eating mindfully can support healthy eating habits.

c. Snacking Smartly: Opt for nutritious snacks such as fruits, vegetables, nuts, and yogurt to satisfy cravings and provide energy throughout the day.

d. Seeking Professional Guidance: Consulting with a registered dietitian or healthcare provider can provide personalized guidance on nutrition and weight management during the postpartum period.

Physical Activity:

a. Gradual Return to Exercise: Engaging in gentle exercises and gradually increasing physical activity can promote overall well, being and assist with weight management. It is important to consult with a healthcare provider before starting any exercise routine, ensuring that the body has adequately healed.

b. Incorporating Physical Activity into Daily Routine: Finding opportunities to be active throughout the day can be beneficial. Taking walks with the baby, practicing yoga or gentle stretching, and incorporating short bouts of physical activity can contribute to overall fitness.

c. Exercise as Self, Care: Viewing exercise as a form of self, care rather than a means for weight loss can promote a positive mindset and a healthy relationship with physical activity.

Emotional Well, being:

a. Self, Compassion: Recognize that the postpartum period is a time of adjustment, and weight loss may not occur as quickly as desired. Be patient with yourself and practice self, compassion. Focus on nurturing your body and mind rather than striving for an unrealistic post, baby body.

b. Mental Health Support: Reach out for emotional support when needed. Postpartum mood disorders can affect self, esteem and body image. Seeking professional help from a therapist or joining support groups can provide the necessary support and guidance.

Building a Supportive Environment:

a. Surrounding Yourself with Positive Influences: Foster a supportive environment by surrounding yourself with loved ones who emphasize your well, being and provide encouragement rather than focusing on physical appearance.

Chapter Four

Healing After a Vaginal Delivery

The Journey to Healing: Navigating Postpartum Recovery After a Vaginal Delivery

The birthing process is a remarkable and transformative experience that brings immense joy and fulfillment to a woman's life. After the delivery of a baby through a vaginal birth, the body undergoes a process of healing and recovery. This postpartum period is a critical time for a woman to prioritize self, care, physical healing, and emotional well, being. Below we will explore the various aspects of healing after a vaginal delivery, providing factual information, practical tips, and insights into postpartum recovery.

Physical Healing:

a. Perineal Soreness and Pain: After giving birth vaginally, it is common to experience perineal soreness, swelling, and discomfort. This area, between the vagina and anus, undergoes stretching and possibly tearing during delivery. To promote healing, practicing good hygiene, using warm water to clean the area, and using peri, bottles or sitz baths can provide relief. Applying ice packs or warm compresses can also help reduce swelling and discomfort.

b. Episiotomy or Tear Healing: In cases where an episiotomy (a surgical cut to widen the vaginal opening) or a tear occurs during delivery, proper wound care is crucial. Keeping the area clean, following healthcare provider instructions for stitches or wound care, and avoiding activities that may strain the perineum, such as heavy lifting or prolonged sitting, can support healing.

c. Urinary and Bowel Function: The urinary and bowel functions may be affected after childbirth. Drinking plenty of water, eating a fiber, rich diet, and practicing good bathroom habits, such as avoiding straining during bowel movements, can help prevent constipation and promote regularity. If urinary incontinence or difficulties persist, seeking guidance from a healthcare provider or pelvic floor therapist can be beneficial.

Rest and Recovery:

a. Prioritizing Rest: Adequate rest is vital for postpartum recovery. The body undergoes significant physical and hormonal changes during childbirth, and rest allows it to heal and replenish energy levels. It is essential to listen to the body's signals and prioritize restful activities such as napping, lying down, and avoiding strenuous physical exertion.

b. Assistance and Support: Enlisting the support of loved ones or hiring a postpartum doula can provide valuable assistance with household chores, caring for the baby, and allowing the mother to focus on rest and recovery.

c. Sleep Hygiene: Establishing healthy sleep habits can enhance postpartum recovery. Creating a conducive sleep environment, practicing relaxation techniques, and developing a consistent bedtime routine can aid in obtaining quality sleep, even with the demands of caring for a newborn.

Emotional Well, being:

a. Emotional Adjustments: The postpartum period can be emotionally challenging as new mothers adjust to their new role and experience hormonal fluctuations. It is essential to communicate openly with loved ones, seek emotional support, and engage in self, care practices that promote mental well, being.

b. Postpartum Depression: Postpartum depression is a common condition that affects many new mothers. It is characterized by feelings of sadness, irritability, and a loss of interest or pleasure in daily activities. Seeking help from healthcare providers, therapists, or support groups is crucial for early diagnosis and appropriate treatment.

Breastfeeding:

a. Establishing a Breastfeeding Routine: If choosing to breastfeed, establishing a breastfeeding routine can support postpartum recovery. Seeking guidance from lactation consultants, attending breastfeeding support groups, and practicing proper latch techniques can enhance the breastfeeding experience.

1b. Nipple Care: Proper nipple care is important to prevent soreness or cracking. Applying lanolin cream, using breast pads for moisture absorption, and ensuring a proper latch can help.

Perineal Care

The Road to Recovery: Nurturing Perineal Care in Postpartum Healing

The postpartum period is a time of adjustment, joy, and physical healing for new mothers. Among the various aspects of postpartum recovery, perineal care holds significant importance. The perineum, the area between the vagina and anus, undergoes tremendous stretching and possibly tearing during childbirth. Proper care and attention to this delicate region can contribute to a more comfortable and efficient healing process. Below we will explore the importance of perineal care, provide factual information, and offer practical tips to support postpartum recovery.

Understanding Perineal Healing:

a. Perineal Soreness and Swelling: After a vaginal delivery, it is common for the perineum to be sore and swollen. This discomfort may last for several days or weeks. The perineum may also exhibit bruising or the presence of stitches in cases of episiotomy or tears. These sensations are normal parts of the healing process and vary from woman to woman.

b. Promoting Healing: Proper perineal care helps promote healing and alleviates discomfort. By maintaining good hygiene, reducing swelling, and preventing infection, the perineum can heal efficiently.

Hygiene Practices:

a. Gentle Cleansing: Keeping the perineum clean is essential for preventing infection and promoting healing. After using the bathroom, gently wash the area with warm water. Avoid using harsh soaps, which can disrupt the delicate pH balance and cause irritation.

b. Patting Dry: After cleansing, pat the perineum dry with a clean, soft towel. Avoid rubbing, as this can cause further irritation.

c. Peri, Bottle/Squirt Bottle: Many women find using a peri, bottle or squirt bottle filled with warm water helpful for cleansing the perineum after urination or bowel movements. This gentle rinsing can provide soothing relief and promote cleanliness.

d. Proper Wiping Technique: When using toilet paper, it is important to wipe from front to back to prevent the spread of bacteria from the anus to the vagina. Use gentle patting motions rather than harsh wiping.

Managing Discomfort:

a. Sitz Baths: Sitz baths, where the perineal area is immersed in warm water, can help reduce swelling and provide soothing relief. This can be done in a shallow basin or with the use of a specialized sitz bath kit. Adding Epsom salts or herbal infusions to the water may further enhance the healing benefits.

b. Cold Compresses: Applying cold packs or ice packs wrapped in a clean cloth to the perineum can help reduce swelling and numb the area, providing temporary relief. Be sure to wrap the cold pack to avoid direct contact with the skin.

c. Pain Relief Measures: Over, the, counter pain relievers, such as acetaminophen or ibuprofen, can be used as directed by a healthcare provider to manage postpartum pain. Consult with a healthcare professional before taking any medication.

Comfortable Sitting and Movement:

1a. Sitting on Soft Surfaces: Sitting on soft cushions or using specialized postpartum seating devices, such as inflatable doughnut, shaped pillows or specially designed cushions, can help alleviate discomfort by reducing pressure on the perineum.

1b. Shifting Positions: Avoid sitting or standing in one position for prolonged periods. Shifting positions, taking short walks, or lying on your side can prevent additional strain on the perineum and encourage blood circulation.

Clothing Choices:

a. Loose, fitting Clothing: Opt for loose, breathable clothing made from soft materials, such as cotton. Avoid tight, fitting jeans or synthetic fabrics, as they can cause irritation and restrict airflow.

Pelvic Floor Health

Empowering Postpartum Recovery: Nurturing Pelvic Floor Health

The postpartum period is a transformative time filled with joy, love, and the challenges of physical recovery. One essential aspect of postpartum recovery that deserves particular attention is pelvic floor health. The pelvic floor, a network of muscles, ligaments, and tissues, plays a vital role in supporting the pelvic organs and maintaining continence. Pregnancy and childbirth can place significant stress on these muscles, leading to various pelvic floor issues. Below we will explore the importance of pelvic floor health in postpartum recovery, provide factual information, and offer practical tips to support a strong and resilient pelvic floor.

Understanding the Pelvic Floor:

a. Anatomy: The pelvic floor refers to a group of muscles that span the area between the pubic bone and the tailbone. These muscles support the bladder, uterus, and rectum, helping to control urinary and bowel functions.

b. Pregnancy and Childbirth Impact: During pregnancy, the weight of the growing baby and hormonal changes can strain the pelvic floor muscles. Vaginal childbirth can further stretch and weaken these muscles. It is not uncommon for women to experience pelvic floor issues postpartum.

Pelvic Floor Issues:

a. Urinary Incontinence: Stress urinary incontinence, characterized by the leakage of urine during activities such as coughing, sneezing, or laughing, is a common pelvic floor issue after childbirth. Hormonal changes and weakened pelvic floor muscles contribute to this condition.

b. Pelvic Organ Prolapse: Pelvic organ prolapse occurs when the pelvic organs (bladder, uterus, or rectum) descend or bulge into the vagina due to weakened pelvic floor muscles. This condition can cause discomfort and impact daily activities.

c. Pelvic Pain: Some women may experience pelvic pain or discomfort after childbirth. This can be due to muscle tension, scar tissue, or other factors related to the pelvic floor.

Pelvic Floor Rehabilitation:

a. Pelvic Floor Exercises: Performing regular pelvic floor exercises, also known as Kegel exercises, can help strengthen the pelvic floor muscles. These exercises involve contracting and relaxing the muscles that control urinary and bowel functions. Consulting a healthcare provider or pelvic floor therapist can provide guidance on proper technique and individualized exercise programs.

b. Breathing and Relaxation Techniques: Deep breathing and relaxation techniques can help release tension in the pelvic floor and promote overall relaxation.

c. Posture and Alignment: Maintaining proper posture and alignment can support pelvic floor health. Avoiding prolonged periods of sitting, maintaining good body mechanics when lifting objects, and practicing good posture throughout the day can alleviate strain on the pelvic floor muscles.

Optimal Bladder and Bowel Habits:

a. Fluid Intake: Adequate hydration is important for overall health and urinary system function. Drinking enough water throughout the day can promote regular urination and prevent urinary tract infections.

1b. Timed Voiding: Establishing a regular voiding schedule can help train the bladder to empty at appropriate intervals, reducing the risk of urinary incontinence.

1c. Avoid Straining: Straining during bowel movements can place unnecessary pressure on the pelvic floor muscles. Consuming a fiber, rich diet, staying hydrated, and practicing good toilet habits, such as avoiding prolonged sitting on the toilet, can promote healthy bowel movements.

Seek Professional Guidance:

a. Pelvic Floor Therapy: If experiencing persistent pelvic floor issues, seeking the guidance of a pelvic floor therapist can be beneficial. These healthcare professionals specialize in the evaluation and treatment of pelvic floor disorders and can provide personalized strategies for recovery.

1b. Healthcare Provider Support: Discussing any concerns about pelvic floor health with a healthcare provider is important.

Chapter Five

Healing After a C, section

Nurturing Recovery: Embracing Healing After a C, Section

The journey of postpartum recovery encompasses a range of physical and emotional changes, and for those who have undergone a cesarean section (C, section) birth, the healing process involves unique considerations. A C, section is a surgical procedure in which a baby is delivered through an incision in the mother's abdomen and uterus. As with any surgical intervention, proper care and attention are vital to ensure a smooth recovery. Below we will explore the importance of healing after a C, section, provide factual information, and offer practical tips to support postpartum recovery.

Understanding C, Section Recovery:

a. Incision Care: The incision made during a C, section requires proper care to prevent infection and promote healing. This incision may be horizontal (low transverse) or vertical (classical or high vertical) depending on the specific circumstances of the birth.

b. Potential Discomfort: After a C, section, it is common to experience discomfort, pain, and fatigue. The recovery process can take several weeks, and each woman's experience may vary.

Managing Incision Healing:

a. Incision Care: Following the healthcare provider's instructions for incision care is crucial. Keeping the incision clean and dry, as well as avoiding excessive bending, stretching, or lifting, can facilitate healing.

b. Managing Pain: Appropriate pain management, as prescribed or recommended by a healthcare provider, can help alleviate discomfort. This may include over, the, counter pain relievers or prescribed medications.

c. Incision Scar Care: After the incision has healed, scar massage or silicone gel sheets may be recommended to help minimize the appearance of the scar and promote tissue healing. Consult with a healthcare provider for guidance on scar care techniques.

Promoting Physical Healing:

a. Rest and Gentle Movement: Adequate rest is essential for post, C, section recovery. Gradually introducing gentle movements, such as short walks, can improve circulation and prevent complications. Avoid strenuous activities until approved by a healthcare provider.

b. Abdominal Support: Wearing an abdominal binder or supportive clothing can provide comfort and gentle compression to the abdominal area, supporting the healing process.

c. Diet and Hydration: Eating a balanced diet rich in nutrients and staying hydrated can support the body's healing process. Adequate hydration and a nutritious diet can aid in tissue repair and overall recovery.

Emotional Well, being:

a. Emotional Support: Emotional well, being plays a crucial role in post, C, section recovery. Connecting with loved ones, seeking emotional support from healthcare providers or support groups, and practicing self, care can contribute to a positive healing experience.

1b. Processing Feelings: It is normal to have a range of emotions after a C, section. Acknowledging and processing these feelings can facilitate emotional healing. Sharing concerns or seeking professional counseling if needed can be beneficial.

Breastfeeding Support:

1a. Positioning and Comfort: Finding comfortable breastfeeding positions that avoid putting pressure on the incision site is important. Experimenting with different positions, using pillows for support, and seeking guidance from lactation consultants can facilitate a positive breastfeeding experience.

b. Lactation Support: Engaging the support of lactation consultants or breastfeeding support groups can provide valuable guidance and encouragement throughout the breastfeeding journey.

Restoring Strength and Fitness:

1a. Gradual Exercise: Engaging in postpartum exercises that are safe and appropriate can help rebuild strength and restore fitness. Begin with gentle exercises, such as Kegels or gentle core exercises, and gradually progress under the guidance of a healthcare provider.

1b. Seeking Professional Guidance: Consulting with a healthcare provider or a postpartum exercise specialist can provide personalized advice and recommendations tailored to individual needs and circumstances.

Incision Care

The Healing Touch: Essential Incision Care for Postpartum Recovery

The postpartum period is a time of immense joy and adjustment as new mothers navigate the path to recovery and caring for their newborn. For women who have undergone a cesarean section (C, section) birth, proper incision care is essential to promote healing and prevent complications. Incision care involves attending to the surgical wound site, keeping it clean, and supporting the body's natural healing process. Below we will explore the importance of incision care in postpartum recovery, provide factual information, and offer practical tips to ensure a smooth healing process.

Understanding the C, Section Incision:

a. Types of Incisions: C, section incisions can be classified as low transverse (horizontal), which is the most common, or vertical (classical or high vertical), used in specific situations. The type of incision is determined based on the circumstances of the birth and the healthcare provider's judgment.

b. Closure Techniques: C, section incisions are typically closed with stitches, staples, or adhesive strips. The choice of closure technique depends on various factors, including the surgeon's preference and the individual's medical condition.

Importance of Incision Care:

a. Promoting Healing: Proper incision care is vital to prevent infection, support wound healing, and minimize scarring. It plays a significant role in the overall recovery process.

b. Reducing Complications: Consistent and appropriate incision care can minimize the risk of complications such as infection, dehiscence (wound reopening), and delayed healing.

General Incision Care Guidelines:

a. Hand Hygiene: Before touching the incision site, always wash your hands thoroughly with soap and water or use hand sanitizer. This helps prevent the introduction of bacteria into the wound.

b. Incision Inspection: Regularly examine the incision site for signs of infection, such as redness, swelling, discharge, or increasing pain. Report any concerns to your healthcare provider.

c. Incision Cleaning: Follow your healthcare provider's instructions for incision cleaning. This may involve gently cleansing the area with mild soap and water or using sterile saline solution.

d. Drying the Incision: After cleaning, pat the incision dry with a clean towel or allow it to air dry. Ensure the area is completely dry before covering it with a dressing or clothing.

Dressing and Wound Care:

a. Dressing Changes: Depending on your healthcare provider's instructions, you may need to change the incision dressing regularly. Follow the recommended schedule and technique to maintain a clean and dry environment.

1b. Wound Protection: Avoid applying excessive pressure or friction to the incision site. Opt for loose, fitting clothing to prevent rubbing and irritation.

1c. Incision Support: Supporting the incision site with a pillow or folded towel when coughing, sneezing, or moving can help reduce discomfort and minimize strain on the incision.

Managing Discomfort:

a. Pain Management: Follow your healthcare provider's recommendations for pain management, which may include over, the, counter pain relievers or prescribed medications. Taking medication as directed can help alleviate discomfort and promote restful recovery.

1b. Applying Heat or Cold: Applying a warm compress or ice pack to the incision area, as advised by your healthcare provider, may help relieve swelling and discomfort. Be sure to protect the incision site with a cloth or towel when using heat or cold therapy.

Signs of Infection:

1a. Recognizing Infection: Watch for signs of infection, including increased redness, warmth, swelling, pus or discharge, foul odor, or a fever. These symptoms require immediate medical attention.

Recovery Timeline

The Road to Recovery: Navigating the Postpartum Healing Timeline

The postpartum period is a transformative and exciting time for new mothers as they embark on the journey of recovery and adjustment. Understanding the recovery timeline is essential for women to navigate the physical and emotional changes that occur during this phase. While every woman's experience may vary, having a general understanding of the postpartum healing process can provide guidance and reassurance. Below we will explore the stages of postpartum recovery, highlighting important milestones and offering practical insights to support women on their healing journey.

The Immediate Postpartum Period:

a. Physical Changes: In the first few hours after birth, the body undergoes immediate changes as it begins to recover. The uterus starts to contract, gradually returning to its pre, pregnancy size, which may cause cramping sensations.

b. Vaginal Bleeding: Lochia, the postpartum vaginal discharge, is experienced during this period. Initially, it is bright red and heavy, resembling a heavy menstrual period. Over time, the bleeding tapers off and transitions from red to pink to white or yellow.

c. Breast Changes: The breasts begin producing colostrum, a nutrient, rich precursor to breast milk. Engorgement, tenderness, and changes in breast size are common during this phase.

The First Week:

a. Physical Recovery: The first week is characterized by ongoing bleeding and the gradual healing of any perineal tears or C, section incisions. Rest and gentle movement are essential during this period to support healing.

b. Hormonal Shifts: Hormonal changes may lead to mood swings and emotional fluctuations commonly known as the "baby blues." It is important to seek emotional support and communicate openly about feelings during this time.

c. Breastfeeding Challenges: Establishing breastfeeding may involve challenges such as engorgement, nipple soreness, and latch difficulties. Working with lactation consultants or seeking breastfeeding support can be beneficial.

Weeks 2 to 6:

a. Physical Healing: By this stage, the uterus continues to shrink, and bleeding gradually decreases. Incisions and tears heal, and any associated discomfort subsides. It is important to maintain good hygiene and continue practicing self, care.

b. Emotional Adjustments: The emotional rollercoaster may continue during this period. It is crucial to communicate feelings and seek support from healthcare providers, family, and friends.

c. Energy and Fatigue: Energy levels may vary, and fatigue is common during this time. Adequate rest, proper nutrition, and light exercise can help manage energy levels and support recovery.

Weeks 6 to 12:

1a. Healing Progress: By this stage, most physical healing is well underway. The uterus is close to its pre, pregnancy size, and bleeding typically stops. Incision scars continue to fade, and any remaining discomfort resolves.

1b. Emotional Well, being: As hormones stabilize, emotional well, being tends to improve. Engaging in activities that promote self, care and connecting with other mothers can be beneficial during this period.

c. Resuming Activities: With healthcare provider approval, gradually resuming regular activities, including exercise and sexual intimacy, can be explored. It is important to listen to the body's signals and take things at a comfortable pace.

Months 3 to 6:

1a. Continued Recovery: The body continues to adjust and heal during this period. Internal healing, such as the restoration of muscle tone and tissue repair, continues.

1b. Emotional Stability: Emotional well, being generally stabilizes, and the baby blues resolve for most women. However, if persistent feelings of sadness or anxiety persist, it is important to seek professional support.

Chapter Six

Emotional Wellness and Mental Health

Nurturing Your Emotional Well, being: Prioritizing Mental Health During Postpartum Recovery

The postpartum period is a time of immense joy and adjustment as new mothers embark on the journey of motherhood. While it is a time filled with love and excitement, it can also bring forth a range of emotional challenges. Understanding the importance of emotional wellness and mental health during postpartum recovery is crucial for the overall well, being of both the mother and the baby. Below we will explore the significance of emotional wellness, shed light on common mental health concerns, and provide practical tips for promoting mental well, being during the postpartum period.

The Emotional Roller Coaster:

a. Hormonal Changes: After giving birth, a woman's hormone levels rapidly fluctuate, which can contribute to mood swings and emotional ups and downs. This period is commonly referred to as the "baby blues."

b. Postpartum Depression: Postpartum depression is a more severe and persistent form of emotional distress. It is characterized by intense feelings of sadness, hopelessness, and a loss of interest or pleasure in activities.

c. Postpartum Anxiety: Postpartum anxiety involves excessive worry, fear, and intrusive thoughts that may interfere with daily functioning and cause significant distress.

The Importance of Emotional Wellness:

a. Bonding with Your Baby: Emotional well, being plays a crucial role in the establishment of a healthy bond between the mother and the baby. Nurturing emotional wellness allows for better connection and communication.

b. Self, Care: Prioritizing emotional well, being enables mothers to take care of themselves, which is essential for their own recovery and ability to care for their baby effectively.

c. Relationship Satisfaction: A mother's emotional well, being significantly impacts her relationships with her partner, family members, and friends. Nurturing emotional wellness fosters healthier relationships and support networks.

Promoting Emotional Wellness:

a. Seeking Support: Reach out to family, friends, and healthcare providers for emotional support. Establishing a strong support system can provide a safe space to share feelings and seek guidance.

b. Self, Reflection and Acceptance: Engage in self, reflection to understand and accept the emotional challenges you may be experiencing. Acknowledge that it is normal to feel overwhelmed and seek help when needed.

c. Rest and Self, Care: Prioritize rest and self, care activities that promote relaxation and rejuvenation. This can include activities such as taking a warm bath, reading, practicing deep breathing exercises, or engaging in hobbies.

Identifying Warning Signs:

1a. Know the Symptoms: Educate yourself about the signs of postpartum depression and anxiety. Be aware of persistent feelings of sadness, anxiety, lack of interest, changes in appetite, sleep disturbances, and thoughts of harming yourself or the baby.

1b. Communicate Openly: Talk openly with your healthcare provider about your emotional well, being during postpartum check, ups. Share any concerns or symptoms you may be experiencing.

c. Partner Support: Encourage your partner to be involved in your emotional well, being. Open and honest communication can help both partners understand and navigate the challenges together.

Professional Support:

1a. Therapy and Counseling: Individual or group therapy can provide a safe and supportive environment to explore and address emotional challenges. Cognitive, behavioral therapy (CBT) and interpersonal therapy (IPT) are effective treatment options.

1b. Medication: In some cases, medication may be prescribed to manage postpartum depression or anxiety. Consult with your healthcare provider to discuss the potential benefits and risks.

1c. Postpartum Support Groups: Joining a postpartum support group allows you to connect with other mothers who are experiencing similar challenges. Sharing experiences and coping strategies can provide a sense of validation and support.

Baby Blues vs. Postpartum Depression

Navigating the Emotional Journey: Baby Blues vs. Postpartum Depression

The postpartum period is a time of immense joy and transition as new mothers adjust to the demands of motherhood. While it is natural to experience a range of emotions during this time, some women may find themselves facing significant emotional challenges. It is important to distinguish between the "baby blues," a common and temporary condition, and postpartum depression, a more severe and persistent form of emotional distress. Understanding the differences between these two conditions is crucial for identifying the appropriate support and treatment. Below we will explore the baby blues and postpartum depression, shedding light on their symptoms, duration, and available interventions to aid women in their postpartum recovery.

The Baby Blues:

a. Symptoms: The baby blues are characterized by mild mood swings, irritability, tearfulness, and feelings of vulnerability. These emotional changes typically occur within the first week after giving birth and may last for a few days to two weeks.

b. Prevalence: The baby blues are a common experience, affecting up to 80% of new mothers. They are believed to be a result of hormonal fluctuations, exhaustion, and adjustment to the new role of motherhood.

c. Duration: The symptoms of the baby blues usually subside on their own within a relatively short period, typically resolving within two weeks postpartum.

Postpartum Depression:

a. Symptoms: Postpartum depression involves more intense and persistent feelings of sadness, hopelessness, and anxiety. Additional symptoms may include loss of interest in activities, changes in appetite and sleep patterns, feelings of guilt or worthlessness, and thoughts of harming oneself or the baby.

b. Prevalence: Postpartum depression affects approximately 10, 20% of new mothers, making it a relatively common condition. It can arise within the first year after giving birth, with symptoms often appearing within the first three months.

c. Duration: Unlike the baby blues, postpartum depression can persist for an extended period if left untreated. Without intervention, symptoms may continue for several months or even longer.

Risk Factors:

a. Personal History: Women with a history of depression, anxiety, or previous episodes of postpartum depression are at a higher risk of developing postpartum depression.

b. Hormonal Factors: Hormonal fluctuations during pregnancy and after childbirth can contribute to emotional instability and increase the risk of postpartum depression.

c. Life Stressors: Factors such as financial difficulties, lack of social support, relationship problems, or a difficult birth experience can contribute to the development of postpartum depression.

Seeking Help and Support:

1a. Self, Assessment: Mothers should be encouraged to monitor their emotional well, being and be aware of any persistent feelings of sadness, hopelessness, or anxiety. Honest self, reflection can help in recognizing the need for support.

1b. Professional Support: Consulting with a healthcare provider or mental health professional is crucial for an accurate diagnosis and appropriate treatment. They can provide guidance and offer interventions tailored to the individual's needs.

c. Social Support: Engaging with a support network, including partners, family, friends, and support groups, can alleviate feelings of isolation and provide practical assistance and emotional validation.

Treatment Options:

1a. Therapy: Psychotherapy, such as cognitive, behavioral therapy (CBT) or interpersonal therapy (IPT), is a common treatment approach for postpartum depression. Therapy can help individuals develop coping strategies, address negative thought patterns, and enhance self, care practices.

1b. Medication: In some cases, medication may be prescribed to manage the symptoms of postpartum depression. Antidepressant medication can be effective when used in conjunction with therapy or other forms of support.

Seeking Help for Postpartum Mood Disorders

The postpartum period is a time of profound changes and adjustments for new mothers. While many women experience joy and fulfillment during this time, others may find themselves grappling with overwhelming emotions and mood disorders. Postpartum mood disorders, such as postpartum depression and anxiety, are common but treatable conditions that require attention and support. Recognizing the signs, understanding the available resources, and seeking help are crucial steps toward postpartum recovery. Below we will explore the importance of seeking help for postpartum mood disorders, providing factual information and practical advice to empower women on their path to healing.

The Prevalence and Impact of Postpartum Mood Disorders:

a. Postpartum Depression: Postpartum depression affects around 10, 20% of women after childbirth and can significantly impact a mother's well, being, her relationship with her baby, and her ability to perform daily activities.

b. Postpartum Anxiety: Postpartum anxiety is another common mood disorder that affects new mothers, characterized by excessive worry, racing thoughts, and heightened anxiety. It can interfere with daily functioning and impact the mother, baby bond.

c. Other Mood Disorders: In addition to depression and anxiety, some women may experience other mood disorders such as postpartum bipolar disorder or postpartum psychosis, which require immediate professional attention.

Recognizing the Signs:

a. Emotional Symptoms: Common emotional symptoms of postpartum mood disorders include persistent sadness, irritability, mood swings, feelings of worthlessness, guilt, or excessive worry and fear.

b. Physical Symptoms: Physical symptoms can manifest as changes in appetite, sleep disturbances, fatigue, or physical discomfort.

c. Behavioral Changes: Women may experience a loss of interest in activities they once enjoyed, withdrawal from social interactions, difficulty bonding with the baby, or thoughts of self, harm.

The Importance of Seeking Help:

a. Validating Your Feelings: Recognize that your feelings are valid and seeking help is not a sign of weakness. Postpartum mood disorders are common and treatable conditions that many women experience.

b. Ensuring Your Well, being: Seeking help is crucial for your own well, being and the well, being of your baby. By addressing your emotional needs, you can better care for yourself and create a nurturing environment for your child.

c. Breaking the Stigma: Seeking help for postpartum mood disorders helps break the stigma surrounding mental health, encouraging open conversations and support networks.

Building a Support System:

1a. Reach Out to Loved Ones: Share your feelings and concerns with your partner, family, and friends. Building a support system of trusted individuals can provide emotional validation and practical assistance.

1b. Professional Support: Consult with healthcare professionals who specialize in postpartum mental health, such as obstetricians, gynecologists, or mental health therapists. They can provide a comprehensive evaluation, diagnosis, and appropriate treatment options.

c. Support Groups: Join local or online support groups specifically designed for women experiencing postpartum mood disorders. Sharing experiences with others who have gone through similar challenges can be comforting and provide valuable insights and coping strategies.

Treatment Options:

1a. Therapy: Psychotherapy, such as cognitive, behavioral therapy (CBT) or interpersonal therapy (IPT), is often recommended for postpartum mood disorders. Therapy can help identify negative thought patterns, develop coping skills, and improve overall well, being.

1b. Medication: In some cases, medication may be prescribed to manage symptoms. Antidepressants or anti, anxiety medications, when prescribed and monitored by a healthcare professional, can be effective in alleviating symptoms and aiding recovery.

Chapter Seven

Breastfeeding and Lactation

Breastfeeding is a natural and beautiful aspect of motherhood, providing numerous benefits to both the baby and the mother. Beyond its nutritional value, breastfeeding promotes bonding, boosts the baby's immune system, and aids in postpartum recovery for the mother. Below we will explore the importance of breastfeeding and lactation in the context of postpartum recovery. We will delve into the benefits, challenges, and available resources to help mothers navigate this intimate and rewarding journey.

The Benefits of Breastfeeding:

a. Optimal Nutrition: Breast milk is a complete source of nutrition for infants, offering the ideal balance of nutrients, antibodies, and hormones necessary for their growth and development.

b. Bonding and Emotional Connection: The act of breastfeeding promotes skin, to, skin contact and fosters emotional bonding between the mother and the baby, enhancing their relationship and creating a sense of security.

c. Health Benefits for the Baby: Breast milk provides antibodies that protect infants against various illnesses and infections, reducing the risk of respiratory infections, gastrointestinal disorders, allergies, and chronic diseases later in life.

d. Health Benefits for the Mother: Breastfeeding can aid in postpartum recovery by reducing the risk of postpartum bleeding, promoting uterus contraction, and assisting in weight loss. It also lowers the risk of breast and ovarian cancer, type 2 diabetes, and cardiovascular disease for the mother.

Challenges of Breastfeeding:

a. Initial Adjustments: In the early days, establishing breastfeeding can be challenging as both the mother and the baby navigate the learning process. Common challenges include latching difficulties, nipple soreness, engorgement, and finding a comfortable position.

b. Milk Supply Concerns: Some women may worry about their milk supply, especially in the early weeks. It is important to remember that milk production is supply and demand, based, and the baby's frequent feeding stimulates milk production.

c. Time and Commitment: Breastfeeding requires time and dedication. It can be demanding, especially during the first few weeks when frequent feeding is necessary. Mothers may need to adjust their routines and find support to prioritize breastfeeding.

Support and Resources:

a. Healthcare Professionals: Seek guidance from lactation consultants, midwives, or nurses who specialize in breastfeeding support. They can provide education, assistance with proper latch techniques, and address any concerns or difficulties.

b. Supportive Networks: Connect with local breastfeeding support groups, either in, person or online, where experienced mothers share their experiences, tips, and encouragement. Peer support can provide invaluable emotional support and practical advice.

1c. Online Resources: Utilize reputable online resources, such as breastfeeding websites, blogs, and forums, for evidence, based information, troubleshooting tips, and guidance on common breastfeeding challenges.

Self, Care and Well, being:

1a. Proper Nutrition: A breastfeeding mother needs a well, balanced diet to meet her nutritional needs and support milk production. Focus on consuming a variety of fruits, vegetables, whole grains, lean proteins, and healthy fats.

b. Hydration: Stay hydrated by drinking an adequate amount of water throughout the day. Breastfeeding can increase thirst, so keep a water bottle nearby and drink whenever you feel thirsty.

1c. Rest and Self, Care: Prioritize rest and self, care to support your physical and emotional well, being. Seek assistance from family and friends to allow for moments of rest and relaxation.

Addressing Challenges:

1a. Seeking Professional Help: If you encounter significant breastfeeding difficulties or concerns, seek help from a lactation consultant or breastfeeding specialist. They can provide personalized support and strategies to overcome challenges.

Establishing a Healthy Milk Supply

Breastfeeding is a remarkable journey that not only provides optimal nutrition for your baby but also offers a unique bonding experience between mother and child. Establishing a healthy milk supply is essential for successful breastfeeding and plays a vital role in postpartum recovery. Below we will explore the importance of establishing a healthy milk supply, address common concerns, and provide practical tips to support lactation and enhance the breastfeeding experience.

Understanding Milk Production:

a. Supply and Demand: Breast milk production operates on the principle of supply and demand. The more the baby feeds, the more milk the body produces to meet the demand.

b. Colostrum: In the initial days after birth, your body produces colostrum, a nutrient, rich and concentrated form of breast milk. It is crucial for your baby's immune system and provides essential nutrients.

c. Mature Milk: Around 3, 5 days after birth, mature milk comes in, which is thinner and more plentiful than colostrum. This milk provides optimal nutrition for your growing baby.

Factors That Influence Milk Supply:

a. Frequent Nursing: The more often your baby nurses, the more milk your body produces. Newborns typically feed 8, 12 times a day, and as they grow, feeding patterns may change.

b. Effective Latch: A proper latch ensures that your baby effectively removes milk from the breast. Seek assistance from a lactation consultant if you encounter difficulties with latching.

c. Emptying the Breasts: It is important to ensure that the breasts are adequately drained during each feeding. Encourage your baby to nurse from both breasts to stimulate milk production.

Tips for Establishing a Healthy Milk Supply:

a. Skin, to, Skin Contact: Practice skin, to, skin contact with your baby soon after birth and during feedings. This promotes bonding, regulates body temperature, and enhances breastfeeding success.

b. Nurse on Demand: Respond promptly to your baby's hunger cues and offer the breast whenever they show signs of hunger. This helps establish a strong milk supply and ensures that your baby receives adequate nutrition.

c. Stay Hydrated and Well, Nourished: Drink plenty of fluids, especially water, to maintain hydration. Eat a balanced diet rich in fruits, vegetables, whole grains, and protein to provide the necessary nutrients for milk production.

1d. Rest and Relaxation: Prioritize rest and relaxation as they are crucial for your overall well, being and milk production. Ensure you get enough sleep, and take breaks throughout the day to rest and recharge.

1e. Avoid Supplementing with Formula: In the early weeks, it is essential to exclusively breastfeed to establish a robust milk supply. Avoid introducing formula unless medically necessary as it can interfere with milk production.

f. Breast Compression: During nursing, gently compress the breast to encourage milk flow and help the baby extract milk effectively. This technique can be especially helpful for babies who may be sleepy or have difficulty nursing.

1g. Pumping and Storing Milk: If you need to be separated from your baby or want to build a milk supply, consider pumping and storing breast milk. Follow proper storage guidelines to ensure its freshness and safety.

Overcoming Common Challenges:

1a. Engorgement: Engorgement occurs when the breasts become overly full and firm, making it difficult for the baby to latch. Apply warm compresses, gently massage the breasts, and nurse frequently to relieve engorgement.

1b. Low Milk Supply Concerns: If you are concerned about low milk supply, consult with a lactation consultant or breastfeeding specialist who can assess the situation and provide guidance tailored to your needs.

1c. Seeking Support: Reach out to support networks such as breastfeeding support groups, lactation consultants,

Overcoming Breastfeeding Challenges

Breastfeeding is a beautiful and natural way to nourish and bond with your baby. However, it is not always a smooth journey, and many mothers encounter challenges along the way. Overcoming these challenges is crucial for both the baby's well, being and the mother's postpartum recovery. Below we will explore common breastfeeding challenges and provide practical tips for overcoming them, ensuring a successful and fulfilling breastfeeding experience.

Latching Difficulties:

a. Seek Assistance: If you're experiencing difficulties with latching, reach out to a lactation consultant or breastfeeding specialist. They can assess the latch and offer guidance on techniques to improve it.

b. Positioning: Experiment with different nursing positions, such as the cradle hold, cross, cradle hold, or football hold, to find the one that works best for you and your baby. Proper positioning can facilitate a better latch.

c. Nipple Care: Ensure your nipples are healthy and moisturized. Apply lanolin cream or nipple butter after each feeding to prevent dryness and soreness.

Engorgement:

a. Frequent Nursing: Breastfeed your baby frequently to prevent engorgement. The more often you empty your breasts, the less likely you are to experience excessive fullness and discomfort.

b. Gentle Massage and Warm Compresses: Use gentle massage and warm compresses to relieve engorgement. Massage your breasts in a circular motion before nursing, and apply warm compresses to encourage milk flow.

c. Cold Compresses: If engorgement persists, apply cold compresses or ice packs after nursing to reduce swelling and discomfort.

Low Milk Supply:

a. Increase Frequency and Duration of Feedings: Offer the breast more frequently and allow your baby to nurse for longer periods. This helps stimulate milk production and increases your milk supply.

b. Pumping and Breast Compression: After nursing, pump to stimulate additional milk production. You can also use breast compression techniques during nursing to enhance milk flow.

c. Proper Nutrition and Hydration: Maintain a healthy diet and stay hydrated to support milk production. Consume foods rich in lactogenic properties, such as oatmeal, fenugreek, and fennel.

Sore Nipples:

1a. Correct Latch: Ensure your baby is latched properly, with their mouth covering both the nipple and a portion of the areola. A correct latch reduces the likelihood of nipple soreness.

1b. Nipple Care: Apply lanolin cream or nipple butter after each feeding to soothe and protect sore nipples. Air, dry your nipples whenever possible to promote healing.

c. Breast Milk Application: Express a small amount of breast milk and gently rub it on your nipples. Breast milk has natural healing properties that can aid in the recovery of sore nipples.

Mastitis and Blocked Ducts:

1a. Empty the Breast: Ensure that your breasts are fully emptied during each feeding. If you suspect a blocked duct, nurse more frequently on the affected side and apply warm compresses before nursing.

1b. Massage and Heat: Massage the affected area gently, moving toward the nipple, to help clear the blockage. Applying a warm compress or taking a warm shower can also promote milk flow.

1c. Rest and Self, Care: Get plenty of rest and take care of yourself. Mastitis often occurs when a mother is exhausted or rundown, so prioritize self, care to support your overall well, being.

Seeking Support:

1a. Join Support Groups: Connect with other breastfeeding mothers through local support groups or online communities. Sharing experiences and advice can provide valuable support and encouragement.

1b. Reach Out to Professionals: Don't hesitate to seek guidance from lactation consultants, midwives, or breastfeeding specialists.

Chapter Eight

Physical Activity and Exercise

Welcoming a new baby into the world is a transformative experience for any mother. Along with the joy and fulfillment, the postpartum period brings physical changes and the need for recovery. Engaging in physical activity and exercise can play a vital role in postpartum recovery, helping mothers regain strength, improve well, being, and promote overall health. Below we will explore the importance of physical activity and exercise in the postpartum period, providing guidance on safe and effective practices.

Benefits of Physical Activity and Exercise:

a. Physical Recovery: Engaging in appropriate exercises can aid in the recovery process by strengthening muscles, promoting circulation, and restoring pelvic floor function.

b. Mental Well, being: Physical activity releases endorphins, promoting feelings of happiness and reducing symptoms of postpartum depression and anxiety.

c. Weight Management: Regular exercise can assist in shedding pregnancy weight and returning to pre, pregnancy fitness levels.

d. Energy Boost: Despite the exhaustion that often accompanies new motherhood, physical activity can actually increase energy levels and combat fatigue.

Consultation with Healthcare Provider:

Before embarking on any exercise regimen, it is essential to consult with your healthcare provider. They can assess your specific postpartum needs, evaluate any complications from delivery, and provide personalized recommendations for physical activity.

Early Postpartum Period:

a. Rest and Recovery: In the immediate postpartum period, the focus should primarily be on rest and recovery. Allow your body time to heal before engaging in more strenuous activities.

b. Gentle Movement: Incorporate gentle movement into your routine, such as walking or gentle stretching exercises, to promote blood circulation and prevent muscle stiffness.

c. Pelvic Floor Exercises: Perform gentle pelvic floor exercises, such as Kegels, to strengthen the pelvic floor muscles and support bladder control.

Gradual Progression:

As your body heals and gains strength, you can gradually increase the intensity and duration of your physical activities. Here are some guidelines to follow:

a. Start Slowly: Begin with low, impact exercises, such as swimming, yoga, or Pilates, that focus on core strength and flexibility.

b. Listen to Your Body: Pay attention to your body's signals. If an activity causes pain, discomfort, or excessive fatigue, modify or decrease the intensity.

1c. Posture and Alignment: Focus on maintaining good posture and proper body alignment during exercises to prevent injury and maximize benefits.

1d. Incremental Increases: Gradually increase the duration and intensity of your workouts. Allow your body time to adapt and recover between sessions.

Pelvic Floor Exercises:

a. Importance of Pelvic Floor: The pelvic floor muscles undergo significant stress during pregnancy and childbirth. Pelvic floor exercises can help restore strength and function.

1b. Kegel Exercises: Practice Kegel exercises regularly to strengthen the pelvic floor muscles. Contract and hold the muscles for a few seconds before releasing. Gradually increase the duration and repetitions.

1c. Incorporate Pelvic Floor Exercises: Incorporate pelvic floor exercises into your daily routine, such as during feeding sessions or while waiting in line.

Supportive Gear:

Investing in supportive gear, such as a supportive bra and comfortable workout clothes, can enhance comfort and provide necessary support during physical activity.

Finding Time for Exercise:

1a. Prioritize Self, Care: Make self, care a priority and schedule dedicated time for exercise. Enlist the help of a partner, family member, or caregiver to watch the baby while you engage in physical activity.

1b. Incorporate Baby into Exercise: Include your baby in your exercise routine. Use a baby carrier or stroller for walks or join postnatal exercise classes specifically designed for mothers and babies.

Safe Postpartum Exercises

The postpartum period is a time of physical recovery and adjustment for new mothers. Engaging in safe and appropriate exercises during this phase can have numerous benefits, including improving strength, promoting mental well, being, and enhancing overall postpartum recovery. Below we will explore the importance of safe postpartum exercises and provide guidelines for a gradual and effective return to physical activity.

Understanding the Postpartum Body:

After childbirth, a woman's body goes through significant changes. It is crucial to understand these changes and respect the body's healing process before embarking on any exercise routine.

a. Hormonal Changes: Hormonal fluctuations, such as decreased estrogen and progesterone levels, can affect ligaments and joints, requiring caution during exercise.

b. Abdominal Separation: Diastasis recti, a condition characterized by the separation of the abdominal muscles, is common after pregnancy. Specific exercises can help repair this separation.

c. Pelvic Floor Healing: The pelvic floor muscles, which support the uterus, bladder, and rectum, undergo stress during childbirth. Exercises to strengthen and restore the pelvic floor are essential.

Timing and Clearance from Healthcare Provider:

Before initiating any postpartum exercise program, it is crucial to consult with your healthcare provider. They can evaluate your specific situation, assess any complications or conditions, and provide clearance for safe exercise.

Early Postpartum Exercises:

During the initial weeks after childbirth, focus on gentle movements that aid in the body's recovery and encourage blood circulation.

a. Walking: Start with short walks around the house or outdoors, gradually increasing the duration as tolerated. Walking not only promotes physical activity but also provides a mental boost.

b. Deep Breathing and Gentle Stretching: Incorporate deep breathing exercises to promote relaxation and gentle stretching to relieve muscle tension and stiffness.

c. Pelvic Floor Exercises: Begin with gentle pelvic floor exercises, such as Kegels, to activate and strengthen the pelvic floor muscles. Focus on proper technique and gradually increase the intensity.

Gradual Progression:

As the body heals and gains strength, gradually increase the intensity and duration of the exercises. Here are some important considerations:

a. Core Strengthening: Engage in exercises that focus on strengthening the core, including the abdominal muscles, back muscles, and pelvic floor. Start with gentle abdominal bracing and progress to more advanced exercises as advised by your healthcare provider.

b. Resistance Training: Incorporate resistance training exercises using resistance bands or light weights to build muscle strength. Focus on major muscle groups while maintaining proper form.

c. Cardiovascular Activities: Include low, impact cardiovascular exercises, such as swimming or cycling, to improve cardiovascular fitness. Start with shorter durations and gradually increase the intensity and duration over time.

d. Posture and Alignment: Pay attention to proper body alignment and posture during exercises. Maintain a neutral spine and avoid excessive strain on the joints.

1e. Listen to Your Body: Be mindful of any discomfort, pain, or fatigue during and after exercise. If an activity causes pain or excessive fatigue, modify or discontinue it and consult with your healthcare provider.

Special Considerations:

1a. Diastasis Recti: If you have abdominal separation, focus on exercises that target the deep core muscles, such as pelvic tilts and transverse abdominal contractions. Avoid exercises that strain the abdominal muscles, such as crunches or sit, ups.

b. Pelvic Floor Exercises: Continue with pelvic floor exercises to restore strength and function. Consider seeking guidance from a pelvic floor physiotherapist for specialized exercises and techniques.

1c. Breastfeeding Considerations: If breastfeeding, consider feeding or expressing milk before exercise to minimize breast discomfort.

Regaining Core Strength

The postpartum period is a transformative phase that requires attention to physical recovery, particularly in regaining core strength. Pregnancy and childbirth can significantly impact the core muscles, including the abdominal muscles, pelvic floor, and back muscles. Below we will explore the importance of regaining core strength after pregnancy, discuss the factors that affect core strength postpartum, and provide practical strategies to restore and strengthen the core muscles.

Understanding the Postpartum Core:

During pregnancy, the abdominal muscles undergo stretching and separation to accommodate the growing baby. Additionally, the pelvic floor muscles bear the weight of the uterus and experience stress during childbirth. These changes can result in weakened core muscles, leading to various issues such as back pain, poor posture, and compromised pelvic floor function.

Factors Affecting Core Strength:

Several factors influence the recovery and restoration of core strength after pregnancy:

Hormonal Changes: Hormonal fluctuations, particularly the hormone relaxin, can affect joint stability and lead to increased joint laxity, requiring caution when engaging in core, strengthening exercises.

Diastasis Recti: Diastasis recti, the separation of the abdominal muscles, is common postpartum. It is essential to identify and address this condition before initiating core exercises to prevent further separation and promote proper healing.

Pelvic Floor Dysfunction: Weakness or dysfunction in the pelvic floor muscles can occur after childbirth, leading to issues such as urinary incontinence and pelvic organ prolapse. Restoring pelvic floor strength is crucial for overall core stability.

Strategies to Regain Core Strength:

Posture Awareness: Correcting posture is the foundation of core strength. Practice maintaining a neutral spine alignment, engaging the abdominal muscles, and lifting the chest while standing, sitting, and performing daily activities.

Pelvic Floor Exercises: Begin with gentle pelvic floor exercises, such as Kegels, to activate and strengthen the pelvic floor muscles. Gradually progress to more advanced exercises, such as bridges and squats, that incorporate pelvic floor engagement.

Diaphragmatic Breathing: Deep, diaphragmatic breathing promotes relaxation and engages the deep core muscles. Practice inhaling deeply, allowing the abdomen to expand, and exhaling fully to activate the core muscles.

Transverse Abdominis Activation: The transverse abdominis (TA) is a deep abdominal muscle that acts as a natural corset. Focus on activating and strengthening the TA by performing exercises such as abdominal bracing, drawing the navel towards the spine.

Gradual Progression: Begin with low, impact exercises and gradually increase the intensity and complexity over time. Incorporate exercises such as pelvic tilts, bird, dogs, and planks to target the core muscles.

Seek Professional Guidance: Consider consulting a physiotherapist or postpartum fitness specialist who can provide personalized guidance and exercises tailored to your specific needs and recovery timeline.

1Incorporate Functional Movements: Integrate functional movements into your exercise routine, such as carrying your baby, lifting, and bending, to engage the core muscles in daily activities.

1Modify High, Impact Activities: Avoid high, impact exercises and activities that place excessive stress on the pelvic floor and abdominal muscles, such as running or jumping, until you have rebuilt sufficient core strength.

Practice Mindful Movement: Focus on the mind, body connection while performing exercises, paying attention to proper form, alignment, and engaging the appropriate muscles. Avoid compensatory movements that can strain other body parts.

1Consistency and Patience: Restoring core strength takes time, and progress may vary for each individual.

Chapter Nine

Sexual Health and Intimacy After Childbirth

The postpartum period is a time of immense change, both physically and emotionally, for new parents. While the focus is often on the recovery of the body and caring for the newborn, it is essential to address the topic of sexual health and intimacy after childbirth. This chapter explores the impact of childbirth on sexual health, common challenges faced by couples, and practical strategies to nurture and restore intimacy during the postpartum period.

Understanding the Impact of Childbirth on Sexual Health:

Childbirth brings about significant changes to a woman's body, and these changes can affect sexual health and intimacy. Here are some key considerations:

Physical Recovery: The body requires time to heal after childbirth, including the healing of any perineal tears or C, section incisions. Hormonal changes, such as decreased estrogen levels, can also affect vaginal lubrication and elasticity.

Fatigue and Sleep Deprivation: The demands of caring for a newborn can lead to sleep deprivation and exhaustion, impacting both physical and emotional well, being. Fatigue can diminish libido and hinder sexual desire.

Emotional Adjustments: The emotional rollercoaster of new parenthood, coupled with hormonal fluctuations, can affect mood and emotional well, being. Feelings of overwhelm, anxiety, or postpartum depression may influence sexual desire and intimacy.

Common Challenges Faced by Couples:

Navigating the postpartum period can present several challenges to sexual health and intimacy. Some common issues include:

Fear and Anxiety: Concerns about pain, physical changes, or the impact of sexual activity on breastfeeding or the newborn's wellbeing can create anxiety and fear around engaging in sexual intimacy.

Body Image Concerns: Many women experience body image issues after childbirth, feeling self, conscious about weight gain, stretch marks, or changes in breast size. These concerns can affect self, esteem and confidence in intimate situations.

Lack of Desire: Reduced libido or a decrease in sexual desire is common during the postpartum period due to hormonal changes, fatigue, or emotional factors. This can create a disconnect between partners and lead to frustration or tension.

Vaginal Dryness and Discomfort: Hormonal changes postpartum can cause vaginal dryness, making sexual intercourse uncomfortable or painful. This can impact a couple's ability to engage in sexual activity and may require additional lubrication or medical intervention.

Strategies to Nurture Sexual Health and Intimacy:

Open Communication: Establish a safe and open line of communication with your partner, discussing feelings, concerns, and desires related to sexual intimacy. Sharing thoughts and emotions can help build trust and foster understanding.

Patience and Understanding: Recognize that each individual's postpartum recovery journey is unique. Practice patience and understanding, allowing time for physical healing, emotional adjustments, and the gradual return of sexual desire.

1Engage in Non, sexual Intimacy: Intimacy is not limited to sexual activity. Focus on nurturing emotional connections through cuddling, hugging, kissing, and gentle touch. Engaging in non, sexual acts of intimacy can strengthen the bond between partners.

1Incorporate Sensate Focus: Sensate focus exercises involve non, sexual touch and exploration of each other's bodies to enhance intimacy and reconnect on a physical level. These exercises can help reduce anxiety and rebuild trust and comfort.

Seek Professional Guidance: If challenges persist or become a source of significant distress, consider seeking support from a healthcare professional or therapist specializing in postpartum sexual health. They can provide guidance, address concerns, and offer strategies for overcoming obstacles.

Resuming Sexual Activity

The postpartum period is a time of adjustment and recovery for new parents, and one aspect that often requires attention is resuming sexual activity. After childbirth, both physical and emotional changes can impact a couple's sexual relationship. This chapter explores the factors influencing the decision to resume sexual activity, common concerns and challenges, as well as practical strategies to navigate this important aspect of postpartum recovery.

Factors Influencing the Decision to Resume Sexual Activity:

The decision to resume sexual activity after childbirth is deeply personal and varies for each couple. Several factors influence this decision:

Physical Recovery: The body needs time to heal after childbirth, especially in the case of vaginal birth or cesarean section. Physical discomfort or pain may affect a woman's readiness to engage in sexual activity.

Hormonal Changes: Hormonal fluctuations, particularly a drop in estrogen levels, can impact vaginal lubrication and elasticity. These changes may influence a woman's comfort and desire for sexual activity.

Emotional Well, being: The emotional adjustments associated with new parenthood, coupled with fatigue and sleep deprivation, can affect a person's libido and overall emotional well, being. Emotional factors play a significant role in deciding when to resume sexual activity.

Breastfeeding: For breastfeeding mothers, the hormonal changes associated with lactation can affect vaginal lubrication and desire for sexual activity. Concerns about the impact of breastfeeding on sexual activity may also arise.

Common Concerns and Challenges:

Couples may face various concerns and challenges when considering the resumption of sexual activity after childbirth. Some common issues include:

Fear and Anxiety: Anxiety about pain or discomfort during sex, worries about the impact on healing or the baby, and concerns about body image can create fear and anxiety around resuming sexual activity.

Body Image and Self, esteem: Many women experience body image concerns after childbirth, including weight gain, stretch marks, or changes in breast size. These concerns can impact self, esteem and confidence in intimate situations.

Communication and Connection: The demands of caring for a newborn can strain communication and emotional connection between partners. Finding time and energy to reconnect on an intimate level may be challenging.

Fatigue and Time Constraints: The sleep deprivation and exhaustion that often accompany caring for a newborn can leave little time or energy for sexual activity. Fatigue can diminish libido and make it difficult to prioritize intimacy.

Strategies for Navigating Resumption of Sexual Activity:

Open Communication: Open and honest communication is key. Discuss expectations, concerns, and desires with your partner. Sharing feelings and understanding each other's perspectives can help alleviate anxiety and build trust.

1Patience and Understanding: Be patient with yourself and your partner. Recognize that postpartum recovery is a gradual process, and it's essential to listen to your body's cues and respect your emotional readiness.

1Gradual Approach: Take a gradual approach to resuming sexual activity. Start with non, penetrative forms of intimacy, such as cuddling, kissing, and caressing. Allow time for physical healing and emotional adjustment before progressing further.

Engage in Non, sexual Intimacy: Intimacy is not solely about sexual activity. Focus on nurturing emotional connections through non, sexual forms of intimacy, such as holding hands, taking walks together, or sharing quality time.

1Lubrication and Comfort: If vaginal dryness or discomfort is a concern, consider using a water, based lubricant to enhance comfort during sexual activity. It's essential to prioritize your comfort and communicate any discomfort with your partner.

Contraception Options

The postpartum period is a time of adjustment and recovery, and it's essential for new parents to consider contraception options as they navigate their reproductive journey. After childbirth, the body undergoes significant changes, and understanding the various contraception methods available can help individuals make informed decisions about their sexual and reproductive health. This chapter discusses different contraception options suitable for postpartum individuals, considering their efficacy, benefits, and considerations in relation to postpartum recovery.

Barrier Methods:

Barrier methods of contraception create a physical barrier between sperm and the cervix to prevent fertilization. These methods include condoms, diaphragms, and cervical caps. They offer immediate protection and have no hormonal side effects. However, they require consistent and correct use to ensure effectiveness. Barrier methods can be particularly useful in the early postpartum period, allowing individuals time to recover and explore other long, term contraception options.

Hormonal Methods:

Hormonal contraception methods use synthetic hormones to prevent ovulation, thicken cervical mucus, and thin the lining of the uterus. These methods include combined hormonal contraceptives (combination pills, patches, and vaginal rings) and progestin, only methods (progestin, only pills, injections, implants, and hormonal IUDs). Hormonal methods are highly effective when used correctly and have additional benefits, such as regulating menstrual cycles and reducing menstrual pain. However, hormonal methods may not be suitable for individuals who are breastfeeding or have specific medical conditions. It's crucial to consult a healthcare provider to determine the most appropriate hormonal method for postpartum individuals.

Intrauterine Devices (IUDs):

IUDs are small, T, shaped devices inserted into the uterus to provide long, acting reversible contraception. There are two types: hormonal (Mirena, Skyla, and Liletta) and non, hormonal (ParaGard). Hormonal IUDs release progestin, which thickens cervical mucus and thins the uterine lining. Non, hormonal IUDs release copper, creating an inhospitable environment for sperm. IUDs are highly effective, last for several years, and are reversible. They can be inserted shortly after childbirth, including during a postpartum check, up. IUDs are suitable for both breastfeeding and non, breastfeeding individuals. However, they may not be recommended for those with certain uterine conditions or a history of pelvic inflammatory disease.

Progestin, Only Pills:

Progestin, only pills, also known as mini, pills, are oral contraceptives that contain only progestin hormones. They are taken daily and work by thickening cervical mucus, inhibiting ovulation, and thinning the uterine lining. Progestin, only pills are a suitable option for breastfeeding individuals since they do not affect milk supply. However, they require strict adherence to the prescribed schedule and may be less effective if not taken at the same time every day. They may not be suitable for individuals with certain medical conditions or those who prefer a more reliable and long, term contraception method.

Sterilization:

Sterilization is a permanent form of contraception that involves surgical procedures to prevent pregnancy permanently. For women, sterilization is typically performed through tubal ligation, where the fallopian tubes are either cut, sealed, or blocked. For men, vasectomy involves cutting or blocking the vas deferens, the tubes that carry sperm. Sterilization should be considered a permanent decision, and individuals should carefully weigh the pros and cons before undergoing the procedure. It is important to note that sterilization does not provide protection against sexually transmitted infections (STIs).

Chapter Ten

Partner Support and Relationship Changes

The postpartum period is a time of significant transition and adjustment for new parents. It brings forth not only physical and emotional changes but also shifts in relationships and dynamics between partners. Understanding the importance of partner support and being prepared for the potential relationship changes can greatly contribute to a positive postpartum recovery experience. Below we will explore the role of partner support during the postpartum period and discuss the common relationship changes that may arise.

The Role of Partner Support:

Partner support plays a crucial role in a new parent's postpartum recovery. It involves emotional support, practical assistance, and active involvement in parenting responsibilities. Here are some ways in which partners can provide support:

a) Emotional Support: Partners can offer understanding, empathy, and a listening ear. They can validate the new parent's experiences and feelings, creating a safe space for open communication. Expressing love, appreciation, and reassurance can help alleviate stress and anxiety.

b) Practical Assistance: Assisting with household chores, cooking meals, and caring for the baby can alleviate the physical burden on the new parent. Partners can take on shared responsibilities to ensure both individuals have time for self, care and rest.

c) Active Involvement in Parenting: Participating in feeding, bathing, diaper changes, and soothing the baby can foster a sense of teamwork and shared responsibility. Partners can attend medical appointments, engage in baby, related research, and take part in parenting classes together.

Relationship Changes:

The arrival of a baby often brings about changes in the dynamics and intimacy between partners. It is essential to recognize and navigate these changes with open communication and understanding. Here are some common relationship changes that may occur:

a) Shift in Priorities: The focus shifts from being solely a couple to being parents. The demands of caring for a newborn can take precedence, and couples may need to find a new balance between their individual needs and the needs of their child.

b) Sleep Deprivation: Sleepless nights can take a toll on both partners, leading to fatigue, irritability, and potential conflict. Supporting each other by taking turns caring for the baby and finding time to rest can help alleviate these challenges.

c) Intimacy and Sexual Changes: Physical and emotional changes after childbirth can impact intimacy and sexual activity. It is important for partners to have open and honest conversations about their desires, concerns, and expectations. Understanding that physical healing takes time and exploring alternative ways of intimacy can help maintain a strong emotional connection.

d) Communication Challenges: Exhaustion and stress can sometimes affect communication between partners. It is crucial to practice active listening, express emotions constructively, and be patient with each other.

Seeking professional support, such as couples counseling, can be beneficial in navigating any communication challenges.

Strengthening the Partnership:

While adjusting to the demands of parenthood, it is important for partners to proactively nurture their relationship. Here are some strategies for strengthening the partnership:

a) Quality Time: Carving out dedicated time for each other, even if it's just a few minutes a day, can help maintain emotional connection. This can involve sharing meals, going for walks together, or engaging in activities that both partners enjoy.

b) Supportive Communication: Actively listening, validating each other's experiences, and expressing gratitude and appreciation can foster a sense of mutual support and strengthen the emotional bond.

1c) Seeking Outside Support: Engaging in couples' support groups or seeking professional help, such as couples therapy, can provide a safe space to address concerns, learn effective communication strategies, and receive guidance during this transitional period.

Communication and Emotional Support

The postpartum period is a time of significant physical and emotional changes for new parents. As they navigate the joys and challenges of parenthood, effective communication and emotional support become vital components of their postpartum recovery. Below we will explore the importance of communication and emotional support during the postpartum period and how they contribute to a positive recovery experience.

Communication in Postpartum Recovery:

Clear and effective communication between partners during the postpartum period is essential for navigating the challenges and joys that arise. Here are some key aspects of communication to consider:

a) Active Listening: Active listening involves giving your full attention to your partner and truly hearing their thoughts and feelings. It creates an environment of trust and openness, allowing each partner to feel valued and understood.

b) Expressing Needs and Emotions: Openly expressing needs, concerns, and emotions is crucial for both partners. It allows for a deeper understanding of each other's experiences and fosters a supportive and nurturing environment.

c) Problem, Solving: Effective communication involves collaboratively addressing challenges and finding solutions together. By working as a team, partners can find practical ways to support each other and overcome obstacles.

d) Patience and Empathy: The postpartum period can be emotionally and physically demanding. It is important for partners to be patient with each other's struggles and show empathy. Understanding that each person may be experiencing their own set of challenges can lead to increased support and understanding.

Emotional Support in Postpartum Recovery:

Emotional support plays a vital role in the postpartum recovery process. It helps new parents cope with the emotional highs and lows, reduces stress, and fosters a sense of connection. Here are some ways to provide emotional support:

a) Validation and Encouragement: Validating your partner's experiences and emotions can be incredibly comforting. Assure them that what they are feeling is normal and that their efforts as a parent are valued. Offering words of encouragement can boost their confidence and overall well, being.

b) Creating Space for Emotional Expression: Postpartum recovery can be an emotional rollercoaster. Encourage your partner to express their emotions openly and without judgment. Provide a safe and non, judgmental space for them to share their fears, anxieties, or feelings of overwhelm.

c) Sharing the Load: Actively participating in childcare responsibilities demonstrates your commitment to sharing the workload. This support allows your partner to have the necessary time and energy to focus on their own recovery.

d) Practicing Self, Care Together: Self, care is essential for both partners during the postpartum period. Encourage and support each other in taking time for self, care activities, such as exercise, relaxation techniques, or pursuing hobbies. This not only promotes individual well, being but also strengthens the bond between partners.

Seeking Additional Support:

In some cases, additional support may be needed to navigate the complexities of postpartum recovery. It is important to be aware of the available resources and not hesitate to seek outside help when necessary. Here are some options to consider:

a) Professional Support: Postpartum doulas, therapists, or counselors specializing in postpartum mental health can provide guidance and support. They can offer strategies for effective communication, coping with emotional challenges, and building a strong support network.

1b) Support Groups: Joining postpartum support groups can connect you with other parents experiencing similar challenges. These groups provide a safe space to share experiences, seek advice, and receive emotional support from individuals who understand the unique aspects of the postpartum journey.

Navigating Changing Dynamics

The arrival of a new baby brings immense joy and excitement, but it also brings significant changes to the dynamics within a family. Navigating these changing dynamics is an essential part of postpartum recovery. Below we will explore the challenges and strategies for navigating changing dynamics during the postpartum period, with a focus on maintaining healthy relationships, adjusting roles and responsibilities, and fostering a supportive environment for all family members.

Maintaining Healthy Relationships:

The postpartum period can place strain on relationships as couples adjust to their new roles as parents. Here are some strategies for maintaining healthy relationships during this time:

a) Open and Honest Communication: Effective communication is crucial for understanding each other's needs and expectations. Make time to discuss concerns, share emotions, and listen actively to your partner. This fosters a sense of closeness and helps address any challenges that may arise.

b) Quality Time: Carve out quality time for you and your partner, even amidst the demands of caring for a newborn. Whether it's a date night, a walk in the park, or simply enjoying a meal together, prioritizing this time strengthens your bond and reinforces your connection as a couple.

c) Expressing Appreciation: Take the time to express gratitude and appreciation for each other's efforts. Recognize and acknowledge the ways in which your partner supports you and contributes to the family. Small acts of kindness and gestures of appreciation can go a long way in maintaining a healthy and loving relationship.

Adjusting Roles and Responsibilities:

The arrival of a baby often requires a reevaluation of roles and responsibilities within the family. Here are some considerations for adjusting roles and fostering a balanced distribution of responsibilities:

a) Shared Parenting: Embrace the concept of shared parenting, where both partners actively participate in the care of the baby. Encourage open discussions about dividing tasks such as feeding, changing diapers, and soothing the baby. This approach promotes equity and ensures that both partners feel involved and valued.

b) Flexibility and Adaptability: Be flexible and willing to adapt as circumstances change. Recognize that roles and responsibilities may shift over time as you navigate the evolving needs of your child. Embrace the concept of teamwork and support each other in finding solutions that work for your family.

c) Asking for Help: It's important to recognize when you need additional support and to ask for help when necessary. Seek assistance from family, friends, or professional support services to alleviate some of the burdens and maintain a healthy balance.

Fostering a Supportive Environment:

Creating a supportive environment is crucial for the well, being of all family members during the postpartum period. Here are some ways to foster such an environment:

a) Cultivating Empathy and Understanding: Recognize that each family member may be experiencing their own unique challenges and emotions during the postpartum period. Practice empathy and seek to understand each other's perspectives. This helps create a safe and supportive space for everyone.

b) Encouraging Self, Care: Encourage each family member, including yourself, to prioritize self, care. Recognize the importance of taking time for personal well, being, whether it's through relaxation techniques, pursuing hobbies, or engaging in physical activities. Supporting each other in self, care promotes overall family well, being.

c) Building a Support Network: Engage with other parents or support groups to build a network of individuals who understand the challenges of the postpartum period. These connections provide opportunities for sharing experiences, seeking advice, and finding support.

1d) Flexibility and Patience: Understand that the postpartum period is a time of adjustment for everyone. Be patient with yourself and your family members as you navigate the changes and challenges.

Chapter Eleven

Returning to Work Postpartum

The postpartum period is a time of significant physical, emotional, and lifestyle changes for new mothers. One important aspect of this phase is the decision to return to work after having a baby. Returning to work postpartum requires careful consideration and planning to ensure a smooth transition and support the ongoing recovery process. Below we will explore the challenges faced by new mothers when returning to work, strategies for managing this transition effectively, and ways to support postpartum recovery in the workplace.

The Challenges of Returning to Work Postpartum:

Returning to work after having a baby can be accompanied by various challenges. It's essential to acknowledge and address these challenges to support the well, being of new mothers. Some common challenges include:

a) Physical Recovery: The postpartum period is a time of physical healing and adjustment. New mothers may still be experiencing physical discomfort, fatigue, or other postpartum symptoms. Balancing these physical demands with the demands of work can be challenging.

b) Emotional Adjustment: The postpartum period is also characterized by emotional adjustments, including hormonal changes and the transition to motherhood. Feelings of guilt, anxiety, or separation from the baby can make the return to work emotionally challenging for new mothers.

c) Childcare Arrangements: Finding suitable and reliable childcare arrangements is crucial for new mothers returning to work. Navigating this process, such as finding the right caregiver, adjusting to separation from the baby, and managing logistics, can be stressful.

Strategies for Managing the Transition:

To navigate the transition of returning to work postpartum successfully, it's essential to have a well, thought, out plan and utilize effective strategies. Here are some strategies to consider:

a) Planning Ahead: Begin the planning process well in advance. Consider factors such as the desired length of maternity leave, work schedule flexibility, and childcare arrangements. Having a clear plan in place helps reduce anxiety and ensures a smoother transition.

b) Gradual Return: Consider a gradual return to work, such as starting with part, time hours or a phased, in schedule. This approach allows for a smoother transition and gives new mothers time to adjust to the demands of work while still prioritizing their postpartum recovery.

c) Communication: Open and honest communication with your employer is vital. Discuss your needs, concerns, and expectations regarding your return to work. Explore options such as flexible work hours, telecommuting, or modified duties that may support a smoother transition.

d) Building a Support System: Surround yourself with a strong support system both at work and at home. This can include colleagues, supervisors, friends, and family members who understand and support your transition. Seek guidance and support from other working mothers who have gone through a similar experience.

Supporting Postpartum Recovery in the Workplace:

Creating a supportive work environment is crucial for new mothers returning to work postpartum. Employers can take steps to support their employees' postpartum recovery and ensure a smooth transition. Here are some initiatives employers can consider:

a) Flexible Work Options: Provide flexibility in work hours or the ability to work from home, if possible. This flexibility allows new mothers to manage their work responsibilities while accommodating their postpartum recovery needs.

b) Lactation Support: Establish a lactation support program that includes designated nursing spaces, breaks for pumping or breastfeeding, and policies that promote breastfeeding support. This helps new mothers maintain their breastfeeding goals and supports their overall well, being.

1c) Mental Health Support: Recognize the importance of mental health and provide resources for employees to access counseling services, if needed. Create a culture that promotes open dialogue about mental health and offers support without judgment.

Balancing Motherhood and Career

The journey of motherhood is a beautiful and transformative experience. It is a time filled with joy, love, and immense responsibility. However, one of the most significant challenges faced by many new mothers is finding the delicate balance between their role as a caregiver and their professional aspirations. Below we will explore the concept of balancing motherhood and a career, focusing on the postpartum recovery period. We will discuss the challenges faced by new mothers, strategies to foster a harmonious relationship between motherhood and career, and the importance of self, care and support during this time.

The Challenges of Balancing Motherhood and Career:

The postpartum recovery period is a critical time for both physical and emotional healing after childbirth. It is during this phase that new mothers must navigate the demanding responsibilities of motherhood while also managing their professional aspirations. Some common challenges faced by new mothers include:

a) Time Management: Juggling the demands of a newborn, household chores, and professional obligations can be overwhelming. Finding a balance between childcare responsibilities and work commitments becomes crucial.

b) Physical Recovery: Postpartum recovery requires adequate rest and self, care. However, balancing this need with professional responsibilities can be challenging, especially if there is limited maternity leave or pressure to return to work quickly.

c) Emotional Well, being: The postpartum period often brings about a range of emotions, including joy, anxiety, and fatigue. Navigating these emotions while maintaining professional focus can be emotionally taxing.

Strategies for Balancing Motherhood and Career:

To foster a harmonious relationship between motherhood and a career during the postpartum recovery period, it is essential to employ effective strategies. Here are some strategies that can help new mothers navigate this delicate balance:

a) Prioritize and Delegate: Identify priorities and delegate tasks whenever possible. Determine what tasks are most important and focus your energy on those while seeking support from family members, friends, or professional services for other responsibilities.

b) Flexible Work Arrangements: Explore flexible work options, such as flexible hours or telecommuting, if feasible. This allows for greater control over your schedule, facilitating a better balance between childcare and work responsibilities.

c) Set Realistic Expectations: Adjust your expectations regarding productivity and career progression during the postpartum recovery phase. Recognize that it is normal for priorities to shift temporarily, and focus on maintaining a healthy work, life integration rather than striving for perfection in all areas.

d) Effective Time Management: Develop effective time management strategies to make the most of the available hours. Prioritize tasks, create a schedule, and establish boundaries to ensure dedicated time for both motherhood and career, related activities.

The Importance of Self, Care and Support:

During the postpartum recovery period, it is crucial for new mothers to prioritize self, care and seek support. Here are some important aspects to consider:

a) Physical Self, Care: Prioritize self, care activities that promote physical well, being, such as proper nutrition, regular exercise, and adequate rest. Taking care of your physical health directly impacts your ability to handle the demands of motherhood and your career.

b) Emotional Well, being: Acknowledge and address your emotional needs. Seek emotional support from loved ones, participate in support groups for new mothers, and consider counseling or therapy if necessary. Prioritizing your emotional well, being enhances your overall ability to balance motherhood and career.

1c) Establishing Support Systems: Build a network of support that includes family, friends, and other new mothers. Surrounding yourself with individuals who understand the challenges you face can provide encouragement, guidance, and practical help when needed.

Childcare Considerations

The journey of becoming a parent is both exciting and challenging. As new parents navigate the postpartum recovery period, one of the most important considerations is childcare. Finding the right childcare arrangements is crucial for the well, being of both the child and the parents. Below we will explore various childcare considerations in relation to postpartum recovery. We will discuss the importance of childcare, different options available, factors to consider when choosing childcare, and the impact of quality childcare on postpartum recovery.

The Importance of Childcare during Postpartum Recovery:

During the postpartum recovery period, new parents need adequate time to rest, heal, and adjust to their new roles. While the primary focus is on the mother's physical and emotional recovery, both parents require support to ensure a smooth transition into parenthood. Here are some reasons why childcare is essential during this time:

a) Physical Recovery: Childbirth can be physically demanding, and new mothers often require rest and recuperation. Having reliable childcare allows mothers to prioritize their recovery by providing the necessary time for rest, self, care, and healing.

b) Emotional Well, being: The postpartum period can bring about a range of emotions, including joy, exhaustion, and anxiety. Having trusted childcare in place provides parents with peace of mind, allowing them to focus on their emotional well, being and bond with their baby without the added stress of constant caregiving.

c) Balancing Responsibilities: New parents often need to resume their work or other commitments during the postpartum recovery period. Childcare enables parents to fulfill their responsibilities while ensuring their child's well, being.

Childcare Options:

When considering childcare options, it is essential to explore various choices that best align with your family's needs and values. Here are some common childcare options:

a) Family Support: Many families rely on the support of extended family members, such as grandparents or siblings, for childcare assistance. This option can provide a familiar and loving environment for the child while allowing parents to maintain close family connections.

b) In, home Caregivers: Hiring an in, home caregiver, such as a nanny or au pair, provides personalized care within the comfort of your own home. This option offers flexibility and convenience, as the caregiver can tailor their services to the family's specific needs.

c) Childcare Centers: Childcare centers, also known as daycare or nursery schools, offer a structured and social environment for children. They are typically licensed facilities with trained staff members who provide care, education, and socialization opportunities for children of various age groups.

d) Co, operative Childcare: Co, operative childcare involves a group of parents taking turns caring for each other's children. This arrangement allows for shared responsibilities, building a sense of community among parents, and providing childcare at a lower cost.

Factors to Consider when Choosing Childcare:

When selecting childcare, it is crucial to consider several factors to ensure the well, being and safety of your child. Here are some key considerations:

a) Safety and Security: Evaluate the safety measures in place, such as child-proofing, emergency procedures, and staff background checks. Ensure that the childcare environment is secure and meets safety standards.

b) Quality of Care: Assess the caregiver's qualifications, experience, and training. Look for a nurturing and stimulating environment that promotes the child's development, including age, appropriate activities and learning opportunities.

1c) Flexibility and Availability: Consider the operating hours, location, and flexibility of the childcare option. It is important to choose an arrangement that aligns with your schedule and can accommodate any changes that may arise.

Chapter Twelve

Postpartum Check, ups and Health Screenings

The postpartum period is a critical time for a new mother's physical and emotional well, being. While the focus tends to be on caring for the newborn, it is equally important for mothers to prioritize their own health and recovery. Postpartum check, ups and health screenings play a vital role in monitoring and supporting a woman's recovery after childbirth. Below we will explore the significance of postpartum check, ups and health screenings in relation to postpartum recovery. We will discuss the importance of these appointments, the recommended timeline for check, ups, the specific screenings conducted, and the benefits they offer to new mothers.

The Importance of Postpartum Check, ups:

Postpartum check, ups are an essential component of postpartum care. They provide an opportunity for healthcare providers to monitor a woman's physical and emotional well, being, assess any postpartum complications or concerns, and offer guidance and support during the recovery period. Here are some key reasons why postpartum check, ups are crucial:

a) Physical Recovery: Pregnancy and childbirth can have a significant impact on a woman's body. Postpartum check, ups allow healthcare professionals to assess the progress of physical recovery, monitor healing, and address any concerns related to childbirth, related injuries or complications.

b) Emotional Well, being: The postpartum period is a time of emotional adjustment and vulnerability. Postpartum check, ups provide a supportive environment for women to discuss their emotional well, being, including feelings of sadness, anxiety, or postpartum depression. Healthcare providers can offer guidance, resources, and referrals to support mental health during this period.

c) Breastfeeding Support: Postpartum check, ups are an opportunity for healthcare providers to offer guidance and support for breastfeeding. They can address any concerns or challenges related to breastfeeding, provide lactation support, and ensure the infant's nutritional needs are being met.

d) Contraception and Family Planning: Postpartum check, ups offer an opportunity to discuss contraception options and family planning with healthcare providers. This is important for women who wish to space their pregnancies or prevent unintended pregnancies during the postpartum period.

Recommended Timeline for Postpartum Check, ups:

The frequency and timing of postpartum check, ups may vary depending on factors such as the woman's overall health, the type of delivery (vaginal or cesarean), and any complications experienced during childbirth. However, the American College of Obstetricians and Gynecologists (ACOG) recommends the following general guidelines:

a) Within the First 3 Weeks: The initial postpartum check, up typically occurs within the first three weeks after delivery. This visit allows healthcare providers to assess the woman's physical recovery, evaluate any postpartum complications, monitor the healing of the perineum (if applicable), and address immediate concerns.

b) 6, 8 Weeks Postpartum: The next postpartum check, up is usually scheduled around 6, 8 weeks after delivery. This visit provides an opportunity for healthcare providers to assess the woman's overall recovery, including the healing of any cesarean incisions, evaluate emotional well, being, discuss contraception options, and address any long, term concerns.

Health Screenings during Postpartum Check, ups:

In addition to physical assessments and emotional support, postpartum check, ups often include specific health screenings to ensure the well, being of new mothers. Some common health screenings during the postpartum period include:

a) Blood Pressure Measurement: Monitoring blood pressure is essential during the postpartum period, as conditions like preeclampsia can persist or develop after childbirth. High blood pressure can indicate potential health risks and requires appropriate management.

Importance of Follow

,

up Appointments

The postpartum period is a crucial time for a woman's physical and emotional well, being. Following childbirth, it is essential for new mothers to prioritize their recovery and ensure they receive the necessary care and support. One vital aspect of postpartum care is attending follow, up appointments with healthcare providers. Below we will explore the importance of follow, up appointments in relation to postpartum recovery. We will discuss the reasons why these appointments are crucial, the recommended frequency and timing, and the benefits they offer to new mothers.

Monitoring Physical Recovery:

Follow, up appointments provide an opportunity for healthcare providers to monitor a woman's physical recovery after childbirth. Pregnancy and childbirth can take a toll on the body, and it is important to assess the healing process and address any concerns that may arise. During these appointments, healthcare professionals can:

a) Evaluate Healing Progress: Follow, up appointments allow healthcare providers to assess the healing of perineal tears or cesarean incisions, if applicable. They can check for any signs of infection or complications and provide appropriate interventions or referrals.

b) Assess Postpartum Symptoms: Women may experience various postpartum symptoms such as vaginal discharge, breast engorgement, or urinary incontinence. By attending follow, up appointments, women can discuss these symptoms with their healthcare providers, who can provide guidance, reassurance, and necessary treatments.

c) Manage Pain: Follow, up appointments offer an opportunity to address any lingering pain or discomfort associated with childbirth. Healthcare providers can discuss pain management strategies and provide appropriate interventions, such as medication or referrals to physical therapists or specialized providers.

Emotional Well, being and Mental Health:

Postpartum follow, up appointments also play a crucial role in supporting a woman's emotional well, being and mental health. The postpartum period can be challenging emotionally, and women may experience a range of emotions and adjustment difficulties. Follow, up appointments provide a safe space for women to:

a) Discuss Emotional Concerns: Women can openly discuss any emotional challenges they may be facing, such as mood swings, postpartum blues, or postpartum depression. Healthcare providers can offer support, screen for mental health disorders, and provide appropriate referrals for further assessment and treatment if needed.

b) Receive Guidance and Resources: Follow, up appointments offer an opportunity for healthcare providers to provide guidance and resources for managing the emotional challenges of the postpartum period. This may include recommendations for support groups, counseling services, or self, care strategies to promote mental well, being.

Breastfeeding Support and Infant Care:

Follow, up appointments are essential for women who are breastfeeding or need guidance in caring for their newborns. Healthcare providers can offer support and guidance in the following areas:

a) Breastfeeding Challenges: Women may encounter various challenges while breastfeeding, such as latching difficulties, low milk supply, or nipple pain. Follow, up appointments allow healthcare providers to assess breastfeeding progress, offer guidance and solutions to overcome challenges, and refer to lactation consultants if necessary.

b) Infant Care: New mothers may have questions or concerns about infant care, including feeding routines, sleep patterns, or general newborn care. Follow, up appointments provide an opportunity for healthcare providers to address these concerns, offer guidance, and ensure the baby's health and development are on track.

Contraception and Family Planning:

Follow, up appointments offer an ideal time for healthcare providers to discuss contraception and family planning with women who want to space their pregnancies or prevent unintended pregnancies during the postpartum period. During these appointments:

a) Contraceptive Options: Healthcare providers can educate women about various contraceptive methods suitable for the postpartum period, taking into consideration factors such as breastfeeding, medical history, and personal preferences.

Vaccinations and Health Screenings

The postpartum period is a critical time for the health and well, being of both the mother and the newborn. During this phase, it is important to prioritize preventive measures to ensure optimal recovery and safeguard against potential health risks. Vaccinations and health screenings play a vital role in protecting the health of postpartum women and their infants. Below we will explore the importance of vaccinations and health screenings in the context of postpartum recovery. We will discuss the recommended vaccinations and screenings, their benefits, and how they contribute to the overall well, being of mothers and infants.

Vaccinations:

Vaccinations are crucial in preventing infectious diseases that can have severe consequences for both mothers and infants. While pregnant women may receive certain vaccinations during pregnancy, postpartum vaccinations are equally important. The following vaccinations are commonly recommended during the postpartum period:

a) Tetanus, Diphtheria, and Pertussis (Tdap): Tdap vaccination is recommended for postpartum women, ideally within 2 to 12 weeks after delivery.

It protects against tetanus, diphtheria, and pertussis (whooping cough). By receiving the Tdap vaccine, mothers can reduce the risk of transmitting pertussis to their newborns, who are particularly vulnerable to severe complications.

b) Influenza: Influenza vaccination is recommended for postpartum women during the flu season. Influenza can lead to serious illness in pregnant and postpartum women, and vaccination helps protect both the mother and the newborn by reducing the risk of flu, related complications.

c) Other Vaccinations: Depending on individual circumstances, healthcare providers may also recommend vaccinations such as the measles, mumps, rubella (MMR) vaccine or the hepatitis B vaccine. These vaccines protect against highly contagious diseases and help ensure the overall health and well, being of mothers and infants.

Health Screenings:

Health screenings are essential during the postpartum period to identify potential health issues and provide appropriate interventions. These screenings help in early detection, prevention, and treatment of various conditions. The following health screenings are commonly recommended:

a) Postpartum Check, up: A comprehensive postpartum check, up is typically scheduled around 6 weeks after delivery. During this visit, healthcare providers assess the mother's overall health, evaluate the healing process, address any concerns, and provide guidance on postpartum recovery.

b) Blood Pressure Monitoring: Postpartum hypertension is a common condition that can have serious implications for both the mother and the baby. Regular blood pressure monitoring during the postpartum period helps identify and manage hypertension, reducing the risk of complications such as preeclampsia or stroke.

c) Pelvic Examination: Pelvic examinations are performed to assess the healing of perineal tears or cesarean incisions, if applicable. These examinations help identify any complications, such as infection or abnormal healing, and ensure proper postpartum recovery.

d) Pap Smear: Depending on a woman's previous screening history, healthcare providers may recommend a Pap smear to screen for cervical cancer. This test is usually performed at the postpartum check, up or at a later stage, based on individual circumstances.

e) Mental Health Screening: Postpartum mental health screening is crucial to identify and address conditions such as postpartum depression, anxiety, or mood disorders. Mental health screenings help ensure timely support and intervention for women who may be experiencing emotional challenges during the postpartum period.

Benefits of Vaccinations and Health Screenings:

Vaccinations and health screenings in the postpartum period offer numerous benefits to both mothers and infants:

Chapter Thirteen

The Role of a Postpartum Doula

The postpartum period is a critical time of physical and emotional transition for new mothers. It is a time when women require support, guidance, and care as they navigate the challenges and joys of early motherhood. One valuable source of support during this phase is a postpartum doula. Below we will explore the role of a postpartum doula and how their presence can significantly contribute to the postpartum recovery process. We will discuss the importance of emotional and physical support, practical assistance, and educational guidance provided by postpartum doulas.

Understanding Postpartum Recovery:

Postpartum recovery refers to the period of adjustment and healing that a woman experiences after giving birth. It involves physical healing, emotional well, being, and the establishment of a new routine with the baby. While each woman's postpartum experience is unique, many women face similar challenges, such as hormonal changes, fatigue, breastfeeding difficulties, emotional adjustments, and lifestyle adjustments. A postpartum doula plays a vital role in helping women navigate these challenges and promotes a healthy recovery.

Emotional Support:

One of the primary roles of a postpartum doula is to provide emotional support to new mothers. The postpartum period can bring a range of emotions, including joy, exhaustion, anxiety, and vulnerability. A doula offers a nurturing presence, a listening ear, and a non, judgmental space for mothers to express their feelings and concerns. They offer validation and reassurance, helping mothers build confidence and cope with the emotional rollercoaster that often accompanies this phase.

Physical Support:

Postpartum doulas also provide valuable physical support to new mothers. They assist with various tasks that promote healing and comfort. This can include helping with breastfeeding positions and techniques, offering guidance on postpartum exercises, providing massage or relaxation techniques, and ensuring that mothers are practicing proper self, care. By offering physical support, doulas help alleviate physical discomfort and enhance the recovery process.

Practical Assistance:

In addition to emotional and physical support, postpartum doulas offer practical assistance to new mothers. They help with household chores, meal preparation, and caring for older siblings. By taking on these responsibilities, doulas allow mothers to focus on rest, bonding with the baby, and recovering from childbirth. This practical assistance lightens the load for mothers and allows them to prioritize their well, being during the postpartum period.

Breastfeeding Support:

Breastfeeding can be a significant challenge for many new mothers. Postpartum doulas are trained in breastfeeding support and can offer guidance and assistance to establish successful breastfeeding. They can help with positioning, latch techniques, addressing common breastfeeding concerns, and ensuring that the mother and baby have a positive breastfeeding experience. This support significantly contributes to the physical and emotional well, being of both mother and baby.

Educational Guidance:

Postpartum doulas also play an essential role in providing educational guidance to new mothers. They offer evidence, based information on topics such as newborn care, soothing techniques, infant sleep patterns, and postpartum recovery. Doulas can answer questions, address concerns, and provide resources that empower mothers to make informed decisions regarding their own and their baby's well, being. By providing education, doulas help mothers gain confidence and feel supported in their new role.

Promoting Self, Advocacy:

Postpartum doulas encourage new mothers to become advocates for themselves and their babies. They help mothers navigate the healthcare system, ask important questions, and communicate their needs effectively. Doulas empower women to make informed decisions about their postpartum care, ensuring that their unique needs and preferences are respected.

Benefits of Doula Support

The postpartum period is a significant phase in a woman's life, marked by physical and emotional changes as she transitions into motherhood. It is a time when new mothers require support, guidance, and care to navigate the challenges and joys of early parenthood. One invaluable source of support during this time is a doula. Below we will explore the benefits of doula support in relation to postpartum recovery. We will discuss how doulas enhance the physical and emotional well, being of mothers, provide educational guidance, and promote positive birth experiences.

Emotional Support:

One of the primary benefits of doula support during the postpartum period is the provision of emotional support. Doulas offer a nurturing and non, judgmental presence, creating a safe space for mothers to express their feelings and concerns. They listen actively, offer validation, and provide reassurance during the emotional ups and downs that often accompany the postpartum journey. This emotional support helps mothers develop confidence, reduce feelings of isolation, and promote a positive mindset, all of which contribute to a smoother postpartum recovery.

Physical Support:

Doulas also play a crucial role in providing physical support to new mothers. They offer assistance with activities such as breastfeeding, proper positioning, and latch techniques. Doulas can help alleviate discomfort and provide guidance on postpartum exercises that aid in the recovery process. By offering physical support, doulas contribute to the healing of the body, reduce physical discomfort, and enhance the overall well, being of mothers during the postpartum period.

Educational Guidance:

Another significant benefit of doula support is the provision of educational guidance. Doulas are knowledgeable about various aspects of postpartum recovery, newborn care, and self, care practices. They offer evidence, based information, answer questions, and provide resources that empower mothers to make informed decisions about their health and well, being. Doulas educate mothers on topics such as infant feeding, soothing techniques, sleep patterns, and self, care practices. By imparting knowledge, doulas enable mothers to feel more confident and equipped to navigate the challenges of the postpartum period.

Promoting Partner Involvement:

Doulas also play a role in promoting partner involvement during the postpartum period. They work closely with partners to provide support and guidance, ensuring that they are actively involved in the care of both the mother and the newborn. Doulas educate partners on ways to offer emotional support, assist with practical tasks, and promote bonding with the baby. This involvement strengthens the partnership, creates a supportive environment, and allows for a smoother transition into parenthood.

Improved Birth Experience:

The benefits of doula support extend beyond the postpartum period to the birthing process itself. Research has shown that the presence of a doula during labor and delivery results in more positive birth experiences. Doulas provide continuous support, advocating for the mother's wishes and needs, and offering comfort measures. This support helps reduce the likelihood of medical interventions, enhances communication between the mother and healthcare providers, and increases overall satisfaction with the birth experience. A positive birth experience sets the foundation for a smoother postpartum recovery.

Reduced Risk of Postpartum Depression:

Postpartum doulas also contribute to the reduction of postpartum depression and anxiety. By providing emotional support, validating feelings, and addressing concerns, doulas help mothers cope with the emotional challenges that can arise during the postpartum period. Doulas can identify signs of postpartum mood disorders and provide appropriate referrals to mental health professionals if necessary.

Finding the Right Doula

The postpartum period is a transformative and vulnerable time for new mothers. It is a time when they require support, guidance, and care as they navigate the physical and emotional challenges of recovery while caring for their newborn. One invaluable source of support during this time is a doula. Below we will explore the importance of finding the right doula and how their presence can enhance the postpartum recovery process. We will discuss the qualities to look for in a doula, the benefits of a strong doula, client relationship, and the positive impact on postpartum well, being.

Qualities to Look for in a Doula:

When seeking a doula, it is essential to consider certain qualities that will ensure a positive and beneficial experience. First and foremost, a doula should possess compassion and empathy. These qualities allow the doula to understand and connect with the unique needs and emotions of the new mother. Additionally, effective communication skills are crucial for building a strong rapport and establishing trust. A doula who actively listens and communicates clearly will be better equipped to address concerns and provide appropriate support.

Experience and Training:

Another vital factor to consider is the doula's experience and training. While certification is not required, it can indicate a level of professionalism and adherence to recognized standards of practice. Doulas who have received training in childbirth education, breastfeeding support, and postpartum care can offer a wealth of knowledge and guidance. Additionally, prior experience working with postpartum mothers can instill confidence in their ability to provide effective support during the recovery period.

Compatibility and Personal Connection:

Building a strong doula, client relationship is essential for a positive postpartum experience. The mother should feel comfortable and at ease with the chosen doula. Therefore, compatibility and personal connection play a significant role in selecting the right doula. A doula who aligns with the mother's values, beliefs, and preferences can provide more personalized and meaningful support. Trust and open communication are crucial for creating a safe and supportive environment.

Continuity of Care:

Another consideration when choosing a doula is the availability and commitment to continuity of care. Some doulas offer services that extend beyond the immediate postpartum period, providing ongoing support during the early stages of motherhood. This continuity allows for a seamless transition and consistent support during the recovery process. It can also foster a deeper connection and understanding between the doula and the mother.

Benefits of a Strong Doula, Client Relationship:

A strong doula, client relationship can have numerous benefits for the postpartum recovery journey. First and foremost, the presence of a doula provides emotional support and reassurance. The doula can be a source of validation, understanding, and guidance, helping the mother navigate the ups and downs of early motherhood. This emotional support can alleviate feelings of isolation, anxiety, and overwhelm, promoting a positive and resilient mindset.

Practical Assistance:

In addition to emotional support, doulas can offer practical assistance during the postpartum period. They can help with tasks such as newborn care education, breastfeeding support, and light household chores. This practical assistance can alleviate some of the burdens and allow the mother to focus on her recovery and bonding with her baby. By lightening the load, doulas contribute to a smoother and more enjoyable postpartum experience.

Advocacy and Communication:

Doulas also serve as advocates for the mother's needs and preferences. They can facilitate communication between the mother and healthcare providers, ensuring that her voice is heard and her choices are respected. Doulas can help mothers navigate the healthcare system, provide information on available options, and empower them to make informed decisions about their recovery and the care of their baby.

Chapter Fourteen

Creating a Postpartum Care Plan

The postpartum period is a critical phase in a woman's life that requires special attention and care. After giving birth, mothers experience physical and emotional changes as they recover and adjust to their new role. To ensure a healthy and smooth postpartum recovery, it is essential to create a comprehensive postpartum care plan. Below we will explore the importance of a postpartum care plan, the key elements to include, and how it can support a woman's overall well, being during this transformative period.

The Importance of a Postpartum Care Plan:

A postpartum care plan provides structure and guidance during the postpartum period, which can often be challenging and overwhelming. It helps women prioritize their health and well, being, establish routines, and access the necessary support systems. A well, designed care plan ensures that mothers have the resources they need to recover physically, emotionally, and mentally, allowing them to better care for themselves and their newborns.

Elements of a Postpartum Care Plan:

Physical Recovery:

The physical recovery after childbirth is a significant aspect of postpartum care. The care plan should include measures to support physical healing, such as managing pain, caring for perineal stitches (if applicable), and promoting good nutrition and hydration. It may also involve gentle exercises or physical therapy to restore strength and flexibility in the body.

Emotional Well, being:

Postpartum emotional well, being is equally important as physical recovery. The care plan should address strategies to support emotional health, including self, care practices, emotional support systems, and potential signs of postpartum mood disorders. It may involve scheduling regular check, ins with healthcare providers, therapists, or support groups to address any emotional challenges.

Rest and Sleep:

Adequate rest and sleep are crucial for postpartum recovery. The care plan should include strategies to prioritize rest, such as arranging for help with household chores and childcare, establishing a sleep routine, and ensuring a conducive sleep environment. Adequate rest promotes physical healing, boosts energy levels, and supports overall well, being.

Nutrition and Hydration:

Proper nutrition and hydration are essential during the postpartum period to replenish the body and support lactation (if breastfeeding). The care plan should outline a healthy and balanced diet, including foods rich in essential nutrients, hydration strategies, and potential dietary restrictions or considerations for specific health conditions.

Breastfeeding Support:

For mothers who choose to breastfeed, the care plan should incorporate breastfeeding support. This may involve seeking guidance from lactation consultants, attending breastfeeding classes or support groups, and establishing a breastfeeding routine. Supportive measures can include comfortable breastfeeding positions, ensuring proper latch, and addressing common breastfeeding challenges.

Social Support:

Social support plays a vital role in postpartum recovery. The care plan should identify the individuals or support systems available to the mother, such as partners, family members, friends, or support groups. It may involve arranging help with household tasks, childcare, or emotional support to alleviate the burden on the mother and promote overall well, being.

Self, Care:

Self, care is an integral part of postpartum recovery. The care plan should encourage the mother to prioritize self, care activities that promote relaxation, reduce stress, and enhance overall well, being. This can include activities such as taking walks, practicing mindfulness or meditation, engaging in hobbies, or seeking professional help if needed.

Medical Check, ups:

Regular medical check, ups are essential during the postpartum period to monitor the mother's health and address any potential concerns. The care plan should include a schedule for postpartum follow, up appointments with healthcare providers, including obstetricians, midwives, or primary care physicians.

Planning for Physical Recovery

The postpartum period is a unique and transformative time in a woman's life. After giving birth, a woman's body goes through significant changes as it recovers from pregnancy and childbirth. It is crucial to prioritize physical recovery during this phase to promote overall well, being and support a smooth transition into motherhood. Below we will explore the importance of planning for physical recovery during postpartum, discuss key elements to consider, and provide practical tips to support a healthy healing process.

Understanding Postpartum Recovery:

Postpartum recovery refers to the period following childbirth when a woman's body undergoes a series of physical changes as it returns to its pre, pregnancy state. The duration and experience of recovery can vary from woman to woman, depending on factors such as the mode of delivery (vaginal or cesarean), individual health, and support systems in place. Planning for physical recovery is essential to ensure a healthy and successful transition to postpartum life.

Elements of Planning for Physical Recovery:

Rest and Sleep:

Adequate rest and sleep are crucial for physical healing and overall well, being during the postpartum period. It is essential to prioritize rest and create a conducive sleep environment. Arrange for help with household chores, enlist support from family or friends, and establish a sleep routine that allows for sufficient rest. Taking short naps when the baby sleeps can also help replenish energy levels.

Pain Management:

Childbirth can cause various types of pain and discomfort, including perineal soreness, abdominal pain, or incision discomfort in the case of a cesarean birth. Planning for pain management involves discussing pain relief options with healthcare providers, utilizing over, the, counter pain medication (if recommended), and exploring alternative therapies such as warm compresses, sitz baths, or gentle stretches.

Proper Nutrition and Hydration:

A well, balanced diet and adequate hydration are vital for postpartum recovery. Focus on consuming nutritious foods that provide essential vitamins, minerals, and nutrients to support healing and breastfeeding (if applicable). Include a variety of fruits, vegetables, whole grains, lean proteins, and healthy fats in your meals. Stay hydrated by drinking plenty of water throughout the day.

Gentle Exercise and Movement:

Engaging in gentle exercise and movement can help promote physical recovery after childbirth. Consult with your healthcare provider to determine when it is appropriate to start exercising and which activities are safe for you. Gradually incorporate activities such as walking, stretching, or postnatal yoga into your routine to improve circulation, rebuild strength, and alleviate muscle tension.

Pelvic Floor Exercises:

The pelvic floor muscles undergo significant strain during pregnancy and childbirth. Planning for physical recovery includes incorporating pelvic floor exercises into your routine. These exercises help strengthen the pelvic floor muscles, improve bladder control, and promote faster healing. Consult a healthcare provider or pelvic floor specialist for guidance on how to perform these exercises correctly.

Postpartum Massage:

Postpartum massage can be beneficial for physical recovery, relaxation, and stress reduction. Consider seeking the services of a qualified massage therapist experienced in postpartum care. Massage can help relieve muscle tension, promote circulation, aid in hormone regulation, and provide a sense of well, being. Ensure that the massage therapist is knowledgeable about postpartum, specific techniques and precautions.

Supportive Undergarments:

Wearing supportive undergarments can provide comfort and aid in the healing process. Consider investing in postpartum, specific undergarments, such as supportive bras or compression garments, to provide stability and reduce discomfort. These garments can help with breast engorgement, provide support to the abdominal muscles, and aid in incision healing for cesarean births.

Planning for Emotional Well

,

being

The postpartum period is a time of profound emotional changes and adjustment for new mothers. It is a time when women experience a range of emotions, from joy and excitement to stress and anxiety. Planning for emotional well, being during postpartum recovery is crucial to ensure a smooth transition into motherhood and support the overall health and happiness of both the mother and the baby. Below we will explore the significance of planning for emotional well, being, discuss key elements to consider, and provide practical tips to promote a positive postpartum experience.

Understanding Emotional Changes in Postpartum:

The postpartum period is often accompanied by a rollercoaster of emotions. Hormonal fluctuations, sleep deprivation, physical discomfort, and the demands of caring for a newborn can contribute to heightened emotional sensitivity and vulnerability. It is essential to recognize that these emotional changes are a normal part of the postpartum experience and that seeking support and developing strategies for emotional well, being is crucial.

Elements of Planning for Emotional Well, being:

Social Support:

One of the key elements of planning for emotional well, being in postpartum recovery is establishing a strong support system. Reach out to family, friends, or support groups that can provide emotional support, practical assistance, and a listening ear. Having someone to share experiences, offer guidance, and validate feelings can significantly alleviate emotional distress.

Open Communication:

Maintaining open and honest communication with loved ones, including partners, family members, and friends, is vital during the postpartum period. Share your feelings and concerns, discuss expectations, and express any emotional challenges you may be facing. Effective communication fosters understanding and can lead to increased support and empathy from those around you.

Self, Care:

Self, care is crucial for emotional well, being. Taking time for yourself, even in small increments, can make a significant difference in your overall mood and resilience. Engage in activities that bring you joy and relaxation, such as reading, practicing mindfulness or meditation, taking a warm bath, or pursuing a hobby. Prioritize self, care and ensure you have dedicated moments for self, nurturing.

Healthy Lifestyle:

A healthy lifestyle can contribute to emotional well, being. Focus on nourishing your body with nutritious foods, staying hydrated, and getting regular exercise. Physical activity releases endorphins, which promote positive emotions and reduce stress. Prioritize adequate sleep and establish a consistent sleep routine to support emotional balance.

Emotional Expression:

Finding healthy outlets for emotional expression is essential during postpartum recovery. Journaling, talking to a trusted friend or therapist, or joining a postpartum support group can provide an opportunity to express emotions and share experiences. Creating a safe space to process and release emotions can help alleviate feelings of isolation and promote emotional healing.

Recognize and Accept Emotions:

It is essential to recognize that experiencing a wide range of emotions during the postpartum period is normal. Allow yourself to feel and acknowledge these emotions without judgment or guilt. Understand that fluctuations in mood are common and often temporary. If emotions become overwhelming or persistently interfere with daily functioning, seeking professional help is advisable.

Set Realistic Expectations:

Setting realistic expectations for yourself during the postpartum period is crucial for emotional well, being. Understand that the transition to motherhood can be challenging, and it is okay to ask for help or adjust your expectations. Recognize that there will be good days and challenging days, and it is important to be patient and kind to yourself throughout the journey.

Seek Professional Support:

If feelings of sadness, anxiety, or emotional distress persist or intensify, seeking professional support is important. Postpartum mood disorders, such as postpartum depression or anxiety, are common and treatable.

Chapter Fifteen

Managing Family and Visitors

The postpartum period is a time of immense change, adjustment, and vulnerability for new parents. It is a time when families and friends come together to celebrate the arrival of a new baby. While the support and presence of loved ones can be valuable, it is crucial to establish healthy boundaries and manage family and visitor interactions in a way that promotes the well, being of the new parents and supports their postpartum recovery. Below we will explore the importance of managing family and visitors during the postpartum period and provide practical tips for creating a supportive and nurturing environment.

Setting Boundaries:

Setting boundaries is essential for maintaining a sense of control, privacy, and emotional well, being during the postpartum recovery period. It is important to communicate your needs and expectations clearly to your family and visitors. Here are some tips for setting boundaries:

Communicate your preferences: Let your loved ones know your preferences regarding visits, such as the length of visits, specific visiting hours, or designated rest periods. Be open and honest about your need for privacy and alone time with your newborn.

Limit the number of visitors: Consider limiting the number of visitors during the early weeks or months of postpartum recovery. This will give you and your partner ample time to bond with the baby and establish a routine. Gradually increase the number of visitors as you feel comfortable.

Schedule visits: Instead of having an open, door policy, schedule specific visiting hours or days. This allows you to plan your day and ensures that you have sufficient time for rest, feeding, and self, care.

Establish hygiene practices: Encourage visitors to follow proper hygiene practices, such as washing hands before holding the baby and refraining from visiting if they are unwell. This helps protect the newborn from potential infections.

Delegate responsibilities: If you have family or friends who genuinely want to help, delegate specific tasks such as cooking meals, grocery shopping, or running errands. This not only eases your workload but also allows your loved ones to contribute in a meaningful way.

Emotional Support:

While managing family and visitors, it is important to prioritize emotional support for the new parents. The postpartum period can be emotionally overwhelming, and having a supportive network can make a significant difference. Here are some strategies for fostering emotional support:

Open communication: Share your feelings, concerns, and needs with your partner and close family members. Encourage open and honest conversations that promote understanding and empathy.

Seek professional help if needed: If you are experiencing significant emotional distress, such as postpartum depression or anxiety, do not hesitate to seek professional help. Mental health professionals can provide guidance, support, and appropriate interventions.

Surround yourself with a positive support system: Identify friends, family members, or support groups that can offer emotional support and understanding. Connect with other new parents who are going through similar experiences.

Take time for self, care: Self, care is essential for emotional well, being. Find moments for relaxation, engage in activities that bring you joy, and prioritize self, care rituals such as taking a bath, practicing mindfulness, or engaging in hobbies.

Accept help: Allow yourself to accept help from others. It is not a sign of weakness or incapability but rather a recognition of the demands of the postpartum period. Accepting help can alleviate stress and provide you with valuable support.

Respecting Postpartum Recovery:

Visitors should be considerate of the physical and emotional recovery of the new parents. Here are some suggestions for creating a respectful environment:

Setting Healthy Boundaries

The postpartum period is a time of immense joy and adjustment as new parents navigate the challenges and rewards of caring for their newborn. It is a critical phase that requires physical healing, emotional support, and the establishment of healthy boundaries. Below we will explore the importance of setting healthy boundaries during the postpartum recovery period and provide practical strategies for nurturing yourself and promoting your overall well, being.

Understanding Postpartum Recovery:

Postpartum recovery refers to the process of healing and adjustment that occurs in the weeks and months following childbirth. It involves physical changes, emotional transitions, and the development of a new routine as the body and mind adapt to the demands of caring for a newborn. Setting healthy boundaries during this period is crucial to support the recovery process and ensure the well, being of both the new parent and the baby.

The Importance of Boundaries:

Setting boundaries allows new parents to establish a sense of control, prioritize their needs, and protect their physical and emotional health. Here are some reasons why boundaries are important during the postpartum recovery period:

Physical healing: The body undergoes significant changes during pregnancy and childbirth. Setting boundaries helps new parents prioritize rest, adequate nutrition, and self, care, which are essential for physical healing and recovery.

Emotional well, being: The postpartum period can bring a range of emotions, including joy, exhaustion, and vulnerability. Setting boundaries allows new parents to create a safe and nurturing space where they can openly express their feelings, seek support, and protect their emotional well, being.

Relationship dynamics: The arrival of a baby often shifts relationship dynamics. Setting boundaries helps new parents navigate changes in their relationships with their partner, family, and friends, ensuring that their needs and the needs of their baby are met while maintaining healthy connections.

Strategies for Setting Healthy Boundaries:

Setting healthy boundaries during the postpartum period requires effective communication, self, advocacy, and a clear understanding of your needs and limitations. Here are some strategies to help you establish and maintain boundaries:

Communicate openly: Clearly express your needs, expectations, and limitations to your partner, family members, and friends. Share your feelings, concerns, and preferences regarding visitors, help, and daily routines. Effective communication sets the foundation for respectful and supportive relationships.

Prioritize self, care: Recognize that taking care of yourself is crucial for your well, being and your ability to care for your baby. Set aside time for activities that recharge you, such as taking a walk, enjoying a hobby, or practicing self, care rituals. Communicate your self, care needs to your support network and ask for assistance when necessary.

Establish visiting guidelines: Determine guidelines for visitors, such as visiting hours, the number of visitors at a time, and hygiene practices. Communicate these guidelines to your loved ones, ensuring that they understand and respect your boundaries. Remember, it's okay to limit visitors if you feel overwhelmed or exhausted.

Delegate tasks: Seek assistance from your partner, family, or close friends to help with household chores, meal preparation, or baby care. Delegate specific tasks, clearly communicate your expectations, and express gratitude for the support you receive. Delegating responsibilities allows you to focus on your recovery and bonding with your baby.

Protect your personal space: Create a peaceful and comfortable environment within your home where you can rest, breastfeed, and bond with your baby. Establish boundaries around your personal space, whether it's your bedroom, nursing area, or designated quiet zone. Communicate these boundaries to your household members to ensure a respectful and peaceful atmosphere.

Accepting Help Gracefully

The postpartum period is a transformative and often challenging time for new parents. After childbirth, the body undergoes physical changes, and there is a significant adjustment in daily routines. During this phase, accepting help gracefully becomes crucial to support postpartum recovery and the overall well, being of both the parent and the baby. Below we will explore the importance of accepting help gracefully during postpartum recovery and provide insights into the benefits and strategies for embracing assistance.

The Importance of Accepting Help:

Postpartum recovery is a period that requires physical healing, emotional support, and adjustment to the demands of caring for a newborn. Accepting help allows new parents to:

Promote physical recovery: Childbirth takes a toll on the body, and accepting help allows parents to prioritize rest and self, care, aiding in physical healing and rejuvenation.

Manage emotional well, being: The postpartum period can be emotionally challenging. Accepting help eases the emotional burden, reduces stress, and provides opportunities for parents to focus on their mental health and bond with their baby.

Foster bonding with the baby: By accepting help, parents can devote more time and energy to nurturing their relationship with their newborn, creating a strong foundation for future development.

Maintain healthy relationships: Accepting help allows parents to balance their responsibilities and maintain healthy relationships with their partner, family, and friends. It prevents feelings of overwhelm and resentment, fostering positive connections and support systems.

Benefits of Accepting Help:

Accepting help during the postpartum period offers numerous benefits, including:

Enhanced recovery: With support, parents can prioritize their physical recovery by getting adequate rest, proper nutrition, and engaging in self, care practices.

Reduced stress: Sharing responsibilities with trusted individuals alleviates the stress of managing all aspects of postpartum life alone. This can lead to improved mental well, being and a more positive outlook.

Increased confidence: Accepting help provides reassurance and encouragement, boosting parental confidence and easing the transition into new roles and responsibilities.

Connection and community: Accepting help allows parents to forge deeper connections with their support network, creating a sense of belonging and community during this transformative time.

Strategies for Accepting Help Gracefully:

Accepting help gracefully involves recognizing your needs, communicating effectively, and being open to receiving support. Here are some strategies to help you navigate this process:

Identify your needs: Reflect on the areas where you could benefit from assistance. This may include household chores, meal preparation, newborn care, or emotional support. Understanding your needs will help you articulate them to your support network.

1Communicate clearly: Clearly express your needs and expectations to your partner, family members, and friends. Let them know how they can help and the specific tasks or areas where you would appreciate their support. Effective communication ensures everyone is on the same page.

1Be open to offers: Welcome offers of help and be receptive to the kindness and support extended to you. Remember that accepting help does not diminish your capabilities as a parent but strengthens your network and promotes your well, being.

Establish boundaries: While accepting help, it's essential to set boundaries that align with your preferences and comfort level. Clearly communicate your boundaries, such as preferred visiting hours, duration of assistance, or specific tasks you would like to handle independently.

1Express gratitude: Show appreciation and gratitude to those who offer their support. A simple thank you can go a long way in acknowledging their efforts and reinforcing positive relationships.

1Prioritize self, care: Accepting help allows you to prioritize self, care. Use the time and support you receive to engage in activities that replenish your energy, whether it's taking a soothing bath or having a nap.

Chapter Sixteen

Postpartum Nutrition

The postpartum period is a crucial time for new mothers to focus on their nutrition and overall well, being. After childbirth, a woman's body goes through significant changes, and proper nutrition plays a vital role in supporting postpartum recovery, replenishing energy levels, and promoting overall health. Below we will explore the importance of postpartum nutrition, provide insights into the key nutrients needed during this period, and offer practical tips for maintaining a healthy and balanced diet.

Importance of Postpartum Nutrition:

Postpartum nutrition is essential for several reasons:

Physical recovery: The body undergoes significant changes during pregnancy and childbirth. Adequate nutrition provides the necessary nutrients to support tissue healing, repair muscles, and replenish nutrient stores depleted during pregnancy and labor.

Energy replenishment: Caring for a newborn can be physically demanding and exhausting. Proper nutrition helps replenish energy levels, combat fatigue, and provide the stamina required for daily tasks and caring for the baby.

Breast milk production: For breastfeeding mothers, nutrition is crucial for milk production and quality. A well, balanced diet ensures an adequate supply of essential nutrients for the baby's growth and development.

Hormonal balance: Nutrient, dense foods can help regulate hormone levels and support the body's transition back to its pre, pregnancy state. Balanced nutrition can also aid in managing postpartum mood swings and promoting emotional well, being.

Key Nutrients for Postpartum Recovery:

To support postpartum recovery, it is important to focus on consuming nutrient, dense foods that provide the following key nutrients:

Protein: Protein is essential for tissue repair, wound healing, and muscle recovery. Include lean meats, poultry, fish, eggs, legumes, nuts, and seeds in your diet to ensure an adequate intake of protein.

Iron: Iron levels may be depleted after childbirth, especially if there was significant blood loss during delivery. Iron, rich foods such as lean meats, dark leafy greens, fortified cereals, and legumes can help replenish iron stores and prevent anemia.

Calcium: Calcium is important for bone health and milk production. Include dairy products, fortified plant, based milk, leafy greens, and calcium, fortified foods in your diet to meet your calcium needs.

Omega, 3 fatty acids: Omega, 3 fatty acids have anti, inflammatory properties and can support brain health and mood stability. Fatty fish like salmon and sardines, walnuts, chia seeds, and flaxseeds are good sources of omega, 3 fatty acids.

Fiber: Adequate fiber intake helps prevent constipation, a common postpartum issue. Include whole grains, fruits, vegetables, legumes, and nuts in your diet to promote healthy digestion.

1Vitamins and minerals: Maintain a balanced intake of vitamins and minerals, including vitamin C (found in citrus fruits and bell peppers), vitamin

D (from sunlight and fortified foods), and folate (found in leafy greens, citrus fruits, and legumes). Additionally, focus on consuming a variety of colorful fruits and vegetables to ensure a wide range of vitamins and minerals.

Tips for Postpartum Nutrition:

Here are some practical tips to help you maintain a healthy and balanced diet during the postpartum period:

1Stay hydrated: Drink plenty of water throughout the day to stay hydrated, especially if you are breastfeeding. Carry a water bottle with you as a reminder to drink regularly.

Plan and prepare meals: Plan your meals in advance to ensure you have nutritious options readily available. Prepare meals and snacks in batches to save time and ensure you have nourishing options on hand when you are busy caring for the baby.

Healing Foods and Nutrients

The postpartum period is a critical phase for new mothers, as their bodies undergo significant changes and need time to heal and recover after childbirth. Proper nutrition plays a vital role in supporting postpartum recovery by providing essential nutrients that aid in tissue repair, replenish energy levels, and promote overall well, being. Below we will explore the importance of healing foods and nutrients during the postpartum period, highlighting key nutrients and their sources that can support a healthy recovery.

Importance of Healing Foods and Nutrients in Postpartum Recovery:

The postpartum period is a time of physical and emotional transition, and the body requires specific nutrients to support healing and overall well, being. Here are some key reasons why healing foods and nutrients are crucial during postpartum recovery:

Tissue repair: The body undergoes significant changes during childbirth, and adequate nutrition is essential for tissue repair and healing. Nutrients such as protein, vitamins A and C, and zinc are particularly important for collagen formation, which is vital for wound healing and repairing stretched and torn tissues.

Energy replenishment: The demands of caring for a newborn can be physically and emotionally exhausting. Consuming nutrient, dense foods provides the necessary energy to support the mother's daily activities and the energy requirements of breastfeeding.

Hormonal balance: The postpartum period is characterized by fluctuating hormone levels, which can impact mood and emotional well, being. Certain nutrients, such as omega, 3 fatty acids and B vitamins, play a role in hormone regulation and can support a healthy emotional balance during this time.

Breast milk production: For breastfeeding mothers, adequate nutrition is essential to support the production of breast milk and provide optimal nutrition for the baby. Consuming a well, balanced diet ensures an adequate supply of nutrients in breast milk, supporting the baby's growth and development.

Key Healing Foods and Nutrients for Postpartum Recovery:

Protein: Protein is a crucial nutrient for tissue repair and healing. Include lean meats, poultry, fish, eggs, legumes, and dairy products in your diet to ensure an adequate protein intake.

Iron: Iron is necessary for replenishing iron stores after childbirth and preventing anemia. Good sources of iron include lean meats, fortified cereals, leafy greens, legumes, and dried fruits.

Calcium: Calcium is essential for bone health, muscle function, and milk production. Incorporate dairy products, fortified plant, based milk, leafy greens, and calcium, fortified foods into your diet to meet your calcium needs.

Omega, 3 fatty acids: Omega, 3 fatty acids have anti, inflammatory properties and can support overall well, being. Include fatty fish like salmon and sardines, walnuts, chia seeds, and flaxseeds in your diet to obtain omega, 3 fatty acids.

Vitamin C: Vitamin C is important for collagen synthesis and immune function. Citrus fruits, berries, bell peppers, and leafy greens are excellent sources of vitamin C.

1Vitamin A: Vitamin A is essential for tissue repair and immune function. Include foods such as sweet potatoes, carrots, spinach, and eggs to obtain vitamin A.

1Zinc: Zinc is involved in wound healing, immune function, and hormone regulation. Good sources of zinc include lean meats, whole grains, legumes, nuts, and seeds.

Fiber: Adequate fiber intake promotes healthy digestion and prevents constipation, which is common during the postpartum period. Include whole grains, fruits, vegetables, legumes, and nuts in your diet to increase fiber intake.

Meal Planning and Preparation

The postpartum period is a significant time of transition and recovery for new mothers. Along with caring for their newborns, it is crucial for mothers to prioritize their own well, being by nourishing their bodies with healthy, balanced meals. Meal planning and preparation play a key role in ensuring that postpartum mothers have access to nutritious meals while managing their new responsibilities. Below we will explore the importance of meal planning and preparation during the postpartum period and provide practical tips for creating nourishing meals that support postpartum recovery.

The Importance of Meal Planning and Preparation during Postpartum Recovery:

The postpartum period is a time when mothers need to focus on their physical and emotional recovery. Adequate nutrition plays a crucial role in supporting the healing process, replenishing energy levels, and promoting overall well, being. Here are several reasons why meal planning and preparation are essential during the postpartum period:

Nourishing your body: Proper nutrition is vital for replenishing nutrient stores and supporting tissue repair after childbirth. Meal planning allows you to ensure that your meals are balanced and contain a variety of nutrient, dense foods that provide the necessary vitamins, minerals, and macronutrients for recovery.

Time, saving: The demands of caring for a newborn can be overwhelming, leaving little time for meal preparation. By planning your meals in advance, you can save time and avoid the stress of deciding what to eat each day. This allows you to focus your energy on taking care of yourself and your baby.

Balanced meals: Postpartum mothers require a well, balanced diet that includes a variety of food groups. Meal planning enables you to create balanced meals that incorporate lean proteins, whole grains, fruits, vegetables, and healthy fats. This ensures that you receive a wide range of nutrients to support your recovery and overall health.

Increased energy levels: Sleep deprivation and the demands of breastfeeding can leave postpartum mothers feeling fatigued. A well, planned and nutritious diet can help boost energy levels, providing the necessary fuel to navigate the challenges of motherhood.

Emotional well, being: Proper nutrition has a significant impact on mood and emotional well, being. Meal planning and preparation allow you to include foods that support brain health and the production of neurotransmitters that promote positive emotions. This can positively influence your overall mental well, being during the postpartum period.

Tips for Effective Meal Planning and Preparation:

Plan meals in advance: Set aside some time each week to plan your meals. Consider your dietary preferences, nutritional needs, and the availability of ingredients. Create a meal plan that includes a variety of meals for breakfast, lunch, dinner, and snacks.

Include nutrient, dense foods: Ensure that your meals are rich in essential nutrients such as lean proteins, whole grains, fruits, vegetables, and healthy fats. These foods provide the necessary vitamins, minerals, and antioxidants for postpartum recovery.

Batch cooking: Take advantage of your energy and time by preparing larger portions of meals that can be stored and reheated throughout the week. This allows you to have nutritious meals readily available, even on busy days.

Stock up on healthy pantry staples: Keep your pantry stocked with nutritious staples such as whole grains, canned beans, nuts, seeds, and spices.

This ensures that you always have the necessary ingredients to create nourishing meals.

1Utilize freezer, friendly meals: Prepare freezer, friendly meals, such as casseroles, soups, and stews, that can be stored and easily reheated when needed. This is particularly helpful during the early weeks of postpartum recovery when time and energy may be limited.

Chapter Seventeen

Caring for Your Newborn

The arrival of a newborn is a momentous and joyous occasion in a parent's life. Along with the excitement and happiness, it also brings new responsibilities and challenges. During the postpartum recovery period, it is essential to provide your newborn with the utmost care and attention while prioritizing your own physical and emotional well, being. Below we will explore the various aspects of newborn care and how it relates to postpartum recovery. From feeding and sleep to hygiene and bonding, we will provide valuable insights to help you navigate this beautiful journey with confidence.

Feeding:

One of the primary aspects of newborn care is ensuring they receive proper nutrition for healthy growth and development. During the postpartum recovery period, feeding your baby becomes a significant focus. Here are some important considerations for feeding your newborn:

Breastfeeding: Breastfeeding provides numerous benefits for both the mother and the baby. It helps establish a strong bond, provides essential nutrients, and boosts the baby's immune system. It is important to establish a breastfeeding routine and seek guidance from lactation consultants or healthcare professionals if needed.

Bottle, feeding: If you choose to bottle, feed your baby, it is crucial to select the appropriate formula and ensure proper sterilization of feeding equipment. Follow the recommended guidelines for feeding intervals and quantities, and pay attention to your baby's cues for hunger and fullness.

Seeking support: Breastfeeding or bottle, feeding can present challenges for new mothers. It is important to seek support from healthcare providers, lactation consultants, or support groups to address any difficulties or concerns you may have.

Sleep:

Newborns require plenty of sleep for their growth and development. However, their sleep patterns may differ from adults, and establishing healthy sleep habits can be a gradual process. Here are some tips for promoting healthy sleep for your newborn:

Create a soothing environment: Ensure the sleep environment is calm, quiet, and comfortable for your baby. Dim the lights, maintain a moderate temperature, and use gentle white noise or lullabies to create a soothing atmosphere.

Establish a routine: Establishing a consistent bedtime routine helps signal to your baby that it is time to sleep. This can include activities such as a warm bath, gentle massage, reading a bedtime story, or singing a lullaby.

Follow safe sleep practices: Follow safe sleep guidelines recommended by healthcare professionals. Place your baby on their back to sleep on a firm mattress in a crib or bassinet free of blankets, pillows, or stuffed animals.

Nap when your baby naps: The postpartum recovery period can be physically and emotionally demanding. Take advantage of your baby's nap times to rest and recharge, as sleep deprivation can affect your overall well, being.

Hygiene and Diapering:

Maintaining proper hygiene and ensuring your baby's comfort is essential during the postpartum recovery period. Here are some key aspects to consider:

Diapering: Regularly change your baby's diapers to keep them clean and prevent diaper rash. Use gentle wipes or warm water and cotton pads for cleaning. Apply a diaper cream or ointment to protect their skin.

Bathing: Give your baby regular baths using warm water and mild baby soap. Take care to support their head and neck during bath time. Ensure the room is warm and have all necessary supplies ready before starting.

1Cord care: If your baby's umbilical cord stump has not yet fallen off, keep it clean and dry. Follow your healthcare provider's instructions for caring for the umbilical cord until it heals completely.

Understanding Newborn Behavior

Welcoming a newborn into your life is a beautiful and transformative experience. As a new parent, understanding your baby's behavior is key to providing them with the care and support they need during the postpartum recovery period. Below we will explore the fascinating world of newborn behavior and its relation to postpartum recovery. From crying and sleep patterns to feeding cues and social interaction, we will delve into the various aspects of newborn behavior, offering insights to help you navigate this special time with confidence and understanding.

Crying:

Crying is the primary means of communication for newborns. While it can be challenging to decipher the different cries, it is essential to recognize and respond to your baby's needs. Here are some common reasons for crying and tips to address them:

Hunger: Hunger is one of the most common reasons for crying. Look for feeding cues such as smacking lips, rooting, or sucking on fingers, and respond by offering breast or bottle.

Discomfort: Your baby may cry if they are uncomfortable due to wet or soiled diapers, clothing that is too tight, or feeling too hot or cold. Check for these factors and make the necessary adjustments to ensure their comfort.

Sleepiness: Babies often become fussy when they are tired. Create a soothing environment and help them settle into a sleep routine to avoid overtiredness.

Need for attention: Newborns crave human contact and may cry to seek comfort and reassurance. Holding your baby, gentle rocking, or skin, to, skin contact can help provide the emotional support they need.

Sleep Patterns:

Understanding your baby's sleep patterns can help establish healthy sleep habits and promote better rest for both of you. Here are some important points to consider:

Sleep cycles: Newborns have shorter sleep cycles than adults, ranging from 45 minutes to 3 hours. They may wake up frequently during the night for feeding or diaper changes. Be prepared for interrupted sleep and try to rest when your baby sleeps.

Day, night confusion: Newborns often have their days and nights mixed up. To help them adjust, expose them to natural daylight and engage in stimulating activities during the day, while creating a calm and dim environment for nighttime sleep.

Safe sleep practices: Follow safe sleep guidelines recommended by healthcare professionals. Place your baby on their back to sleep, in a crib or bassinet free of blankets, pillows, or stuffed animals.

Feeding Cues:

Recognizing your baby's feeding cues is crucial for timely and adequate nourishment. Here are some common feeding cues to watch for:

Rooting reflex: When a baby turns their head and opens their mouth when you stroke their cheek or mouth, it indicates they are ready to feed.

Hand, to, mouth movements: Babies may suck on their fingers, hands, or fists when they are hungry.

1Smacking lips or tongue movements: These are signs that your baby is preparing to feed.

1Increased alertness or restlessness: Babies may become more alert or fidgety when they are hungry.

It is important to respond promptly to your baby's feeding cues to establish a healthy feeding routine and ensure they receive adequate nutrition for growth and development.

Social Interaction:

Newborns are social beings from the moment they are born. Understanding their social cues and engaging in responsive interactions is vital for their emotional well, being. Here are some key points to consider:

Eye contact: Babies are drawn to human faces and make eye contact as early as a few weeks old. Maintain eye contact with your baby during feeding, diaper changes, and playtime to establish a strong connection.

Baby's Health Check

,

ups

Bringing a new baby into the world is a joyous and transformative experience. As a parent, it is crucial to prioritize your baby's health and well, being during the postpartum recovery period. Regular health check, ups play a vital role in monitoring your baby's growth, development, and overall health. Below we will explore the importance of baby's health check, ups, the recommended schedule, and the various aspects of the check, ups in relation to postpartum recovery.

Why are Baby's Health Check, ups Important?

Regular health check, ups for your baby are essential for several reasons. First and foremost, they allow healthcare professionals to monitor your baby's growth and development, ensuring that they are thriving and meeting important milestones. Regular check, ups also provide an opportunity for healthcare professionals to address any concerns or issues that may arise and provide guidance and support to parents.

Additionally, these check, ups serve as an important opportunity for parents to discuss any questions or concerns they may have about their baby's health, feeding, sleeping, and general well, being. It is an opportunity for parents to gain knowledge, receive guidance, and build a relationship with their healthcare provider.

Recommended Schedule for Baby's Health Check, ups:

The recommended schedule for baby's health check, ups may vary depending on the country or healthcare system. However, a general guideline is as follows:

Newborn Visit (within the first week): Shortly after birth, your baby will have their first health check, up. During this visit, healthcare professionals will assess the baby's overall health, perform physical examinations, and provide guidance on breastfeeding or formula feeding, newborn care, and postpartum recovery for parents.

1, Month Visit: Around one month of age, your baby will have their next check, up. This visit focuses on monitoring growth, evaluating feeding and sleep patterns, and addressing any concerns or questions you may have.

2, Month Visit: At the 2, month mark, your baby will have another check, up. During this visit, healthcare professionals will track your baby's growth, administer vaccinations, and discuss developmental milestones.

4, Month Visit: The 4, month check, up is an important milestone in your baby's health journey. It involves monitoring growth, development, and administering vaccinations.

6, Month Visit: At 6 months, your baby will have another check, up to evaluate their growth, development, and milestones. Healthcare professionals may introduce solid foods during this visit and address any concerns you have regarding your baby's health and well, being.

9, Month Visit: The 9, month check, up focuses on assessing your baby's physical and cognitive development, addressing any concerns, and providing guidance on nutrition, safety, and developmentally appropriate activities.

12, Month Visit: The 12, month check, up is a significant milestone as it marks your baby's first year of life. Healthcare professionals will assess your baby's growth, development, and milestones. Immunizations and important screenings may also be conducted during this visit.

Key Aspects of Baby's Health Check, ups:

Physical Examination: During each check, up, healthcare professionals will conduct a thorough physical examination of your baby. This may include measuring height, weight, and head circumference, assessing heart and lung sounds, checking reflexes, and examining the skin, eyes, ears, and abdomen.

Vaccinations: Immunizations are an integral part of your baby's health check, ups. Vaccinations protect your baby from serious diseases and help build their immune system. Healthcare professionals will administer vaccines according to the recommended schedule.

Chapter Eighteen

Postpartum Hair Loss

Bringing a new life into the world is a miraculous journey filled with joy and wonder. However, along with the joys of motherhood, many women experience a temporary and often alarming side effect known as postpartum hair loss. This shedding of hair can be distressing for new mothers, but it is important to understand that it is a normal part of the postpartum recovery process. Below we will explore the causes of postpartum hair loss, its relationship to postpartum recovery, and effective management strategies to cope with this temporary phase.

Causes of Postpartum Hair Loss:

During pregnancy, many women experience a surge in hormones that promote healthy hair growth. As a result, they often notice thicker and more lustrous hair during this time. However, after giving birth, hormonal changes occur, causing the hair growth cycle to shift. This transition from the growth phase to the resting phase can lead to excessive shedding, commonly known as postpartum hair loss. The exact causes of this phenomenon are still being studied, but it is believed to be primarily influenced by hormonal fluctuations.

Relationship to Postpartum Recovery:

Postpartum hair loss is a common occurrence and is typically experienced by the majority of new mothers. It usually begins around three to six months after giving birth and can continue for several months. While it can be concerning and disheartening, it is important to remember that postpartum hair loss is temporary and part of the body's natural healing and adjustment process. Understanding its relationship to postpartum recovery can help women navigate this phase with more confidence and reassurance.

Managing Postpartum Hair Loss:

While postpartum hair loss cannot be entirely prevented, there are strategies that can help manage the shedding and promote healthy hair growth. Here are some effective management strategies for coping with postpartum hair loss:

Maintain a Healthy Diet: Good nutrition is essential for overall well, being, including healthy hair growth. Eating a balanced diet rich in vitamins, minerals, and proteins can support hair health. Include foods such as fruits, vegetables, lean meats, whole grains, and healthy fats in your diet.

Take Postnatal Supplements: Consult with your healthcare provider about postnatal supplements that can provide essential nutrients for hair health, such as biotin, vitamin D, and omega, 3 fatty acids.

Avoid Hairstyling Practices that Cause Stress on Hair: During the postpartum period, it is advisable to avoid hairstyles that pull or tug on the hair, such as tight ponytails or buns. Opt for loose and gentle hairstyles that do not add additional stress to the hair follicles.

Be Gentle with Hair Care: Handle your hair gently while washing, brushing, and styling. Use a wide, toothed comb or a brush with soft bristles to avoid unnecessary hair breakage. Avoid excessive heat styling and harsh chemical treatments that can further damage the hair.

Practice Stress Management: Stress can contribute to hair loss. Engaging in stress, reducing activities such as exercise, meditation, yoga, and spending time on hobbies can help promote overall well, being, including healthy hair growth.

Seek Support: Talking to other new mothers or joining postpartum support groups can provide emotional support and reassurance during this phase. Sharing experiences and coping strategies can be beneficial in managing postpartum hair loss.

Consult a Healthcare Professional: If you have concerns about excessive hair loss or if the shedding persists beyond a year postpartum, it is advisable to consult a healthcare professional. They can assess your specific situation, rule out any underlying medical conditions, and provide personalized advice and treatment options if necessary.

Understanding Postpartum Hair Loss

Bringing a new life into the world is a remarkable experience, but it also brings about various changes in a woman's body. One common change that many new mothers experience is postpartum hair loss. This temporary shedding of hair can be concerning and disheartening for women, especially when combined with the already demanding nature of postpartum recovery. Below we will explore the causes of postpartum hair loss, its relation to postpartum recovery, and ways to understand and manage this natural process.

Causes of Postpartum Hair Loss:

To understand postpartum hair loss, it's important to know the normal hair growth cycle. Hair follicles go through a growth phase (anagen), a transitional phase (catagen), and a resting phase (telogen), after which hair sheds and new hair starts to grow. During pregnancy, the hormonal changes cause an increased percentage of hair follicles to be in the growth phase, leading to thicker and fuller hair. However, after childbirth, hormone levels drop dramatically, resulting in a shift of hair follicles into the resting phase. This transition leads to excessive shedding, known as postpartum hair loss.

Relationship to Postpartum Recovery:

Postpartum hair loss is a natural part of the postpartum recovery process. It usually begins around three to six months after giving birth and can continue for several months. It's essential to understand that this shedding is temporary and does not indicate a serious health problem. The body is simply readjusting to its pre, pregnancy state. Postpartum hair loss is not experienced by every woman, but it is estimated that around 50% to 90% of new mothers will notice some degree of hair shedding during this time.

Managing Postpartum Hair Loss:

While postpartum hair loss cannot be prevented completely, there are ways to manage and minimize its impact. Here are some tips to help cope with postpartum hair loss:

Be Gentle with Your Hair: Avoid hairstyles that pull or tug on the hair, as they can exacerbate hair loss. Instead, opt for loose hairstyles that put less stress on the hair follicles. Be gentle when washing, brushing, and styling your hair to minimize breakage.

Eat a Balanced Diet: Good nutrition plays a crucial role in promoting healthy hair growth. Include foods rich in vitamins, minerals, and proteins in your diet. Focus on consuming fruits, vegetables, lean proteins, whole grains, and healthy fats to support hair health.

Take Care of Your Scalp: Maintaining a healthy scalp can contribute to healthier hair. Keep your scalp clean and moisturized. Avoid using harsh hair products and opt for gentle shampoos and conditioners that are suitable for your hair type.

Manage Stress: High stress levels can worsen hair loss. Find ways to manage stress through activities such as exercise, meditation, deep breathing, or engaging in hobbies you enjoy. Taking care of your mental and emotional well, being is crucial during the postpartum period.

Consult a Healthcare Professional: If you are concerned about the extent of hair loss or if it persists for an extended period, it is recommended to consult a healthcare professional. They can assess your situation, rule out any underlying medical conditions, and provide appropriate guidance or treatment options if needed.

Give Yourself Time: Remember that postpartum hair loss is a temporary phase. It may take several months for your hair to regain its pre, pregnancy thickness. Be patient and give yourself time to adjust and recover.

Tips to Manage Hair Loss

Bringing a new life into the world is a miraculous experience, but it also comes with a range of physical changes for new mothers. One common change that many women experience during the postpartum period is hair loss. This can be a cause of concern and affect a woman's self, esteem. However, it's important to understand that postpartum hair loss is a normal part of the recovery process and usually resolves on its own. Below we will discuss some helpful tips to manage hair loss during the postpartum period.

Understanding Postpartum Hair Loss:

Postpartum hair loss, also known as postpartum alopecia, is a common occurrence that affects many women after childbirth. During pregnancy, hormonal changes cause an increased percentage of hair follicles to be in the growth phase, resulting in thicker and fuller hair. However, after giving birth, hormone levels return to normal, causing a shift in hair follicles to the resting phase. This transition leads to excessive shedding, which can be distressing for new mothers.

Tip 1: Be Gentle with Your Hair:

To manage postpartum hair loss, it's important to be gentle with your hair. Avoid hairstyles that pull or tug on the hair, such as tight ponytails or buns. These styles can put stress on the hair follicles and lead to further hair loss. Opt for loose hairstyles that allow your hair to breathe and minimize tension. Use a wide, toothed comb or a brush with soft bristles to avoid unnecessary breakage when detangling your hair.

Tip 2: Eat a Balanced Diet:

Proper nutrition plays a crucial role in promoting healthy hair growth. Eating a balanced diet rich in vitamins, minerals, and proteins can help support hair health. Include foods such as fruits, vegetables, lean proteins, whole grains, and healthy fats in your meals. Foods like spinach, salmon, eggs, nuts, and avocados are known to nourish the hair follicles and promote hair growth. Consult a healthcare professional or a registered dietitian for personalized dietary recommendations.

Tip 3: Take Care of Your Scalp:

Maintaining a healthy scalp is essential for healthy hair growth. Keep your scalp clean by washing it regularly with a gentle shampoo. Avoid using harsh hair products that can strip the natural oils from your scalp. Consider using a moisturizing conditioner to keep your hair and scalp hydrated. Massaging your scalp gently can stimulate blood circulation and promote hair growth. Using a wide, toothed comb or your fingertips, gently massage your scalp in circular motions for a few minutes each day.

Tip 4: Avoid Excessive Heat Styling:

Excessive heat styling can damage the hair shafts and worsen hair loss. Limit the use of heat styling tools such as flat irons, curling irons, and blow dryers. When using these tools, always apply a heat protectant spray to minimize damage. Consider embracing natural hairstyles that require less heat styling. If you must use heat, set the tools to the lowest heat setting possible and limit the duration of exposure.

Tip 5: Manage Stress:

Stress can contribute to hair loss, so it's important to find healthy ways to manage stress during the postpartum period. Take time for self, care activities that help you relax and unwind. Engage in activities such as meditation, yoga, deep breathing exercises, or taking walks in nature. Seek support from family and friends, and don't hesitate to ask for help when needed. Taking care of your mental and emotional well, being is crucial for overall health and can positively impact hair growth.

Tip 6: Consider Supplements:

In some cases, taking supplements may help support hair health during the postpartum period. Talk to your healthcare provider before starting any extra supplements.

Chapter Nineteen

Body Image and Self, esteem

Postpartum recovery is a transformative and challenging time for new mothers. While the focus is often on physical healing and caring for the newborn, it is equally important to address the emotional well, being of the mother. One crucial aspect of emotional well, being is body image and self, esteem. The changes that occur during and after pregnancy can have a significant impact on how women perceive their bodies and themselves. Below we will explore the relationship between body image, self, esteem, and postpartum recovery, as well as provide tips for nurturing a positive self, image during this transformative period.

Understanding Body Image and Self, esteem:

Body image refers to an individual's perception of their own physical appearance, including their size, shape, and overall attractiveness. Self, esteem, on the other hand, relates to a person's overall sense of self, worth and value. These two concepts are closely intertwined, as body image can greatly influence self, esteem. During postpartum recovery, women experience various physical changes such as weight fluctuations, stretch marks, and changes in breast size, which can impact their body image and subsequently affect their self, esteem.

The Media and Societal Influences:

It is important to recognize that societal and media influences play a significant role in shaping our perception of the ideal body. Images of celebrities and models with seemingly perfect post, baby bodies can create unrealistic expectations and put pressure on new mothers to bounce back immediately. However, it is essential to understand that every woman's postpartum journey is unique, and comparing oneself to these idealized images is neither realistic nor healthy.

Embracing Your Postpartum Body:

Practice Self, Compassion: Be kind and patient with yourself. Remember that your body has gone through an incredible process of creating and nurturing life. Celebrate and appreciate the amazing things your body has accomplished.

Surround Yourself with Positive Influences: Surround yourself with supportive individuals who embrace body diversity and promote positive self, image. Seek out communities, both online and offline, that celebrate and empower postpartum women.

Focus on Health, Not Weight: Shift your focus from weight loss to overall health and well, being. Engage in activities that nourish your body and mind, such as regular exercise, nutritious eating, and self, care practices. Emphasize feeling strong, energized, and healthy rather than attaining a specific body shape or size.

Practice Mindful Self, Care: Incorporate self, care activities into your daily routine. This can include taking relaxing baths, engaging in hobbies you enjoy, practicing mindfulness or meditation, and seeking professional support if needed. Taking care of your mental and emotional well, being is crucial for fostering a positive body image.

Dress for Comfort and Confidence: Choose clothes that make you feel comfortable and confident in your postpartum body. Opt for styles that flatter your body shape and emphasize your favorite features. Don't be afraid to experiment with different clothing options to find what makes you feel good.

Celebrate Non, physical Attributes: Remember that your worth extends far beyond your physical appearance. Acknowledge and celebrate your non, physical attributes, such as your resilience, nurturing nature, intelligence, and creativity. Engage in activities that boost your self, esteem and remind you of your unique strengths and capabilities.

Seek Support: Surround yourself with a supportive network of friends, family, or a postpartum support group. Sharing your thoughts and feelings with others who are going through or have gone through similar experiences can provide validation, reassurance, and perspective.

Embracing Your Postpartum Body

The postpartum period is a unique and transformative time in a woman's life. It is a period of physical healing, emotional adjustment, and bonding with the newborn. One aspect that many women grapple with during this time is body image. The physical changes that occur during pregnancy and childbirth can often lead to mixed feelings and a complex relationship with one's postpartum body. Below we will explore the importance of embracing and accepting your postpartum body, providing insights and tips to foster self, acceptance and confidence during the postpartum recovery journey.

Understanding Postpartum Body Changes:

Pregnancy and childbirth bring significant changes to a woman's body. It is essential to understand and acknowledge these changes to develop a positive attitude towards your postpartum body. Some common postpartum body changes include:

Weight Fluctuations: During pregnancy, women naturally gain weight to support the growing baby. After childbirth, it is normal for the body to shed some of this weight. However, it may take time for the body to return to its pre, pregnancy shape.

Abdominal Changes: The abdominal muscles stretch to accommodate the growing baby, and after childbirth, they may take time to regain their tone. Some women may also experience diastasis recti, a separation of the abdominal muscles that requires specific exercises for recovery.

Breast Changes: Breastfeeding or not, breasts go through changes during pregnancy and postpartum. They may enlarge, become engorged, and later may change in size and shape.

Stretch Marks: Stretch marks are common and result from the stretching of the skin during pregnancy. They can appear on the abdomen, breasts, thighs, and other areas.

Skin and Hair Changes: Hormonal fluctuations can lead to changes in skin texture, including acne, dryness, or pigmentation. Some women may experience postpartum hair loss or changes in hair texture.

Embracing Your Postpartum Body:

Practice Self, Compassion: Be kind and patient with yourself. Understand that your body has gone through a remarkable journey of creating and nurturing life. Appreciate the strength and resilience of your body.

Shift the Focus: Instead of obsessing over your appearance, shift your focus towards the incredible abilities of your body. Celebrate the miracle of childbirth and the nurturing bond you share with your baby.

Surround Yourself with Positive Influences: Surround yourself with supportive individuals who promote body positivity and self, acceptance. Engage in communities or social media platforms that celebrate postpartum bodies and share empowering stories.

Challenge Unrealistic Expectations: The media often portrays unrealistic images of postpartum bodies, creating pressure to bounce back quickly. Remind yourself that every woman's postpartum journey is different, and there is no universal timeline for recovery.

1Celebrate Small Achievements: Set small, realistic goals for your postpartum body and celebrate each milestone. This could be as simple as getting back into your favorite pair of jeans or participating in an exercise routine that brings you joy.

1Engage in Gentle Exercise: Engaging in gentle exercises, such as walking or postnatal yoga, can support your physical and mental well, being. Focus on activities that make you feel good and help you regain strength and energy.

Practice Mindfulness: Be mindful of your thoughts and self, talk. Challenge negative or critical thoughts about your body and replace them with positive affirmations. Practice gratitude for your body's capabilities and the journey it has undertaken.

1Dress for Comfort and Confidence: Invest in comfortable and stylish postpartum clothing that makes you feel confident and classy.

Coping with Body Image Issues

The postpartum period is a time of immense physical and emotional changes for women. While the focus is often on the care of the newborn, it is crucial to address the body image issues that many women experience during this time. Coping with body image issues is an essential aspect of postpartum recovery, as it can impact a woman's self, esteem, mental well, being, and overall adjustment to motherhood. Below we will explore strategies to cope with body image issues during the postpartum period and foster self, acceptance and self, love.

Understanding Body Image Issues:

Body image issues refer to the negative perceptions and feelings individuals have about their physical appearance. In the context of postpartum recovery, body image issues can arise due to the physical changes that occur during pregnancy and childbirth. Some common body image concerns experienced by women during this time include:

Weight and Shape: Many women feel pressure to regain their pre, pregnancy weight and shape quickly. The reality is that it takes time for the body to recover and readjust after childbirth.

Stretch Marks and Scars: Stretch marks and scars can appear on the abdomen, breasts, and other areas as a result of the skin stretching during pregnancy. Some women may feel self, conscious about these marks.

Breast Changes: Breasts often change in size, shape, and firmness during pregnancy and breastfeeding. Some women may struggle with feelings of dissatisfaction or insecurity about their breasts' appearance.

Abdominal Changes: The abdominal area undergoes significant changes during pregnancy, including muscle separation and a loss of muscle tone. Many women may feel self, conscious about their postpartum belly.

Hair and Skin Changes: Hormonal fluctuations can lead to changes in hair texture, thickness, and even hair loss. Skin changes such as acne, pigmentation, and dryness can also impact a woman's body image.

Coping Strategies for Body Image Issues:

Practice Self, Compassion: Be gentle with yourself and practice self, compassion. Recognize that your body has gone through an incredible journey of creating life and that it will take time to adjust and recover.

Surround Yourself with Support: Seek support from loved ones, friends, or support groups who can provide encouragement, understanding, and reassurance. Share your feelings and concerns with people who will uplift and support you.

Challenge Unrealistic Expectations: Reject the societal pressure to "bounce back" immediately after childbirth. Remind yourself that every woman's postpartum journey is unique, and it is normal for bodies to change during and after pregnancy.

Focus on Health and Well, being: Shift the focus from appearance to overall health and well, being. Emphasize self, care activities that promote physical and mental wellness, such as nutritious eating, regular exercise, and sufficient rest.

1Engage in Positive Self, Talk: Challenge negative thoughts and replace them with positive affirmations. Remind yourself of the incredible strength and resilience your body has shown in bringing new life into the world.

1Set Realistic Goals: Set realistic and achievable goals for yourself, taking into consideration your body's needs and limitations. Celebrate each milestone and progress, no matter how small.

Embrace Postpartum Fashion: Invest in comfortable and stylish clothing that makes you feel confident and comfortable in your postpartum body. Choose outfits that flatter your shape and make you feel good about yourself.

1Practice Mindfulness and Body Acceptance: Engage in mindfulness practices that allow you to be present and accepting of your body as it is in the present moment.

Chapter Twenty

Incontinence and Bladder Control

The postpartum period is a time of immense joy and adjustment as women navigate the physical and emotional changes that come with childbirth. While the focus is often on caring for the newborn, it is important to address the issue of incontinence and bladder control, which is a common concern during postpartum recovery. Incontinence refers to the involuntary loss of urine, and it can significantly impact a woman's quality of life and self, confidence. Below we will explore the causes of incontinence, its relation to postpartum recovery, and effective management strategies to regain bladder control.

Understanding Incontinence and its Causes:

Incontinence can manifest in various forms, including stress incontinence, urge incontinence, and mixed incontinence. Stress incontinence occurs when there is a leakage of urine during activities that put pressure on the bladder, such as sneezing, coughing, or lifting. Urge incontinence, on the other hand, is characterized by a sudden and strong urge to urinate, leading to leakage before reaching the restroom. Mixed incontinence is a combination of both stress and urge incontinence.

During the postpartum period, incontinence is primarily attributed to the strain placed on the pelvic floor muscles during pregnancy and childbirth. The pelvic floor muscles support the bladder, uterus, and bowel, and they can become weakened or stretched during pregnancy, especially with vaginal delivery. The hormonal changes and increased pressure on the pelvic floor can result in reduced bladder control.

Effective Management Strategies for Incontinence:

Pelvic Floor Exercises: Pelvic floor exercises, also known as Kegel exercises, are a key component of managing incontinence. These exercises involve contracting and relaxing the pelvic floor muscles to improve their strength and coordination. Regular and correct practice of pelvic floor exercises can help regain bladder control.

Seek Professional Guidance: Consult a healthcare provider or a pelvic floor physiotherapist who specializes in postpartum care. They can provide personalized guidance on pelvic floor exercises, assess the severity of incontinence, and recommend additional treatments or interventions if necessary.

Maintain a Healthy Weight: Excess weight can put additional strain on the pelvic floor muscles and worsen incontinence. Maintaining a healthy weight through balanced nutrition and regular exercise can help alleviate symptoms.

Stay Hydrated: It may seem counterintuitive, but staying properly hydrated can actually help manage incontinence. Adequate hydration maintains the health of the bladder and prevents irritation that can exacerbate symptoms. However, avoid excessive fluid intake close to bedtime to minimize nighttime bathroom visits.

Practice Bladder Training: Bladder training involves gradually increasing the time between bathroom visits to train the bladder to hold larger volumes of urine. Start with small increments and gradually increase the duration between voiding. This can help improve bladder capacity and reduce the frequency of urination.

Use Absorbent Products: During the recovery period, it may be helpful to use absorbent products such as pads or protective underwear to manage any leakage. This can provide a sense of security and minimize any potential embarrassment or anxiety related to incontinence.

Monitor and Modify Dietary Habits: Certain foods and beverages can irritate the bladder and worsen incontinence symptoms. These include caffeine, spicy foods, acidic fruits, and carbonated drinks. Pay attention to your body's response to different foods and consider making adjustments to your diet as needed.

Avoid Straining during Bowel Movements: Straining during bowel movements can put pressure on the pelvic floor muscles and worsen incontinence.

Understanding Postpartum Incontinence

The postpartum period is a time of significant physical and emotional changes for women as they recover from childbirth and adjust to their new roles as mothers. One common issue that many women face during this time is postpartum incontinence, which refers to the involuntary loss of urine after giving birth. While it is a common condition, it can have a significant impact on a woman's quality of life and self, esteem. Below we will explore the causes of postpartum incontinence, its relation to postpartum recovery, and effective management strategies to regain bladder control.

Understanding Postpartum Incontinence:

Postpartum incontinence is a type of urinary incontinence that occurs after childbirth. It can manifest in various forms, including stress incontinence, urge incontinence, or a combination of both. Stress incontinence is the most common type and involves leakage of urine during activities that put pressure on the bladder, such as coughing, sneezing, laughing, or lifting heavy objects. Urge incontinence, on the other hand, is characterized by a sudden and intense urge to urinate, leading to leakage before reaching the restroom.

Causes of Postpartum Incontinence:

Postpartum incontinence is primarily attributed to the changes that occur in the pelvic floor muscles during pregnancy and childbirth. The pelvic floor muscles, which provide support to the bladder, uterus, and bowel, can become weakened or stretched during pregnancy and delivery. The weight of the growing fetus, hormonal changes, and the stretching of the pelvic floor muscles during childbirth can all contribute to postpartum incontinence.

Additionally, vaginal deliveries, especially those involving the use of forceps or vacuum extraction, can increase the risk of pelvic floor trauma and subsequent incontinence. Factors such as obesity, multiple pregnancies, and a history of incontinence prior to pregnancy can also increase the likelihood of experiencing postpartum incontinence.

Postpartum Recovery and Incontinence:

The postpartum recovery period is crucial for addressing and managing postpartum incontinence. While the focus is often on caring for the newborn, it is essential for women to prioritize their own recovery and seek appropriate treatment for incontinence. Ignoring the issue or assuming it will resolve on its own can prolong the condition and negatively impact a woman's physical and emotional well, being.

Effective Management Strategies:

Pelvic Floor Exercises: Pelvic floor exercises, also known as Kegel exercises, are a cornerstone of managing postpartum incontinence. These exercises involve contracting and relaxing the pelvic floor muscles to strengthen and tone them. Regular and consistent practice of pelvic floor exercises can help improve muscle strength and restore bladder control.

Seek Professional Help: Consulting a healthcare provider or a pelvic floor physiotherapist can provide valuable guidance and support in managing postpartum incontinence. They can assess the severity of the condition, provide personalized advice on pelvic floor exercises, and recommend additional treatments if necessary.

Maintain a Healthy Weight: Excess weight can put additional pressure on the pelvic floor muscles, exacerbating incontinence symptoms. Adopting a healthy lifestyle that includes a balanced diet and regular exercise can contribute to weight management and improve overall bladder control.

Stay Hydrated: Adequate hydration is essential for maintaining bladder health. It is important to drink enough water throughout the day to support proper urinary function. However, it is advisable to avoid excessive fluid intake before bedtime to reduce nighttime bathroom visits.

Manage Bowel Function: Constipation can worsen postpartum incontinence as straining during bowel movements can put pressure on the pelvic floor muscles.

Effective Management Strategies

The postpartum period is a transformative and delicate time for new mothers as they navigate the physical, emotional, and hormonal changes that accompany childbirth. It is crucial for women to prioritize their own recovery during this phase to promote overall well, being and ensure a smooth transition into motherhood. Below we will explore effective management strategies for postpartum recovery that encompass both physical and emotional aspects of healing. These strategies aim to support women in their journey towards optimal health and adjustment to their new roles.

Physical Recovery Strategies:

Rest and Sleep:

One of the most important aspects of postpartum recovery is getting sufficient rest and sleep. Sleep deprivation can have a profound impact on a mother's physical and mental well, being. It is recommended to prioritize sleep whenever possible by establishing a consistent sleep routine, taking naps during the day, and seeking help from a partner or support network to share the responsibilities of caring for the newborn.

Nutrition and Hydration:

Proper nutrition is vital for postpartum recovery. A well, balanced diet rich in nutrients can help replenish the body's resources, support healing, and provide the energy needed to care for a newborn. It is important to include a variety of fruits, vegetables, whole grains, lean proteins, and healthy fats in the diet. Adequate hydration is equally essential, as it promotes optimal physical function and helps prevent common postpartum issues like constipation.

Gentle Exercise:

Engaging in gentle exercises can contribute to postpartum recovery by improving blood circulation, rebuilding strength, and boosting mood. It is crucial to consult with a healthcare provider before starting any exercise regimen and gradually increase the intensity as the body heals. Activities such as walking, yoga, and postpartum, specific exercise programs can be beneficial for both physical and emotional well, being.

Pelvic Floor Exercises:

The pelvic floor muscles undergo significant changes during pregnancy and childbirth, and they play a crucial role in postpartum recovery. Performing pelvic floor exercises, also known as Kegel exercises, can help strengthen and tone these muscles, reducing the risk of urinary incontinence and promoting faster healing. It is recommended to consult with a healthcare provider or a pelvic floor physiotherapist for proper instruction and guidance.

Emotional Recovery Strategies:

Seek Support:

Building a strong support network is essential for emotional well, being during the postpartum period. Surrounding oneself with understanding and supportive individuals can provide reassurance, guidance, and an outlet for expressing concerns and emotions. This network may include partners, family members, friends, and healthcare professionals.

Open Communication:

Maintaining open and honest communication with loved ones and healthcare providers is crucial for emotional recovery. Expressing feelings, concerns, and challenges can help alleviate stress and promote understanding and support. Regularly communicating with a partner about emotional needs and sharing responsibilities can also foster a stronger bond and sense of shared responsibility.

Self, Care:

Self, care plays a significant role in postpartum recovery. Taking time for oneself, engaging in activities that bring joy and relaxation, and prioritizing personal well, being can have a positive impact on emotional health. This may include taking soothing baths, practicing mindfulness or meditation, engaging in hobbies, or seeking professional help if needed.

Join Support Groups:

Participating in postpartum support groups can provide a sense of community and a safe space to share experiences and concerns with other new mothers. These groups offer an opportunity to connect with women who are going through similar experiences, share advice, and seek guidance from healthcare professionals specializing in postpartum care.

Chapter Twenty-One

Postpartum Thyroid Issues

The postpartum period is a time of immense change and adjustment for new mothers. While most attention is focused on physical recovery and caring for the newborn, it is important to address the potential impact of hormonal changes on maternal health. One common issue that can arise during this time is postpartum thyroid dysfunction. Below we will explore the relationship between postpartum recovery and thyroid issues, shedding light on the causes, symptoms, and management strategies for this condition.

Understanding Postpartum Thyroid Dysfunction:

Postpartum thyroid dysfunction refers to abnormal thyroid function that occurs in the months following childbirth. There are two main types of thyroid dysfunction that can manifest during this time: postpartum thyroiditis and postpartum Graves' disease.

Postpartum Thyroiditis:

Postpartum thyroiditis is a condition characterized by inflammation of the thyroid gland. It typically occurs in the first year after delivery and is thought to result from an autoimmune response triggered by the hormonal changes associated with pregnancy. Initially, the condition may present with hyperthyroidism, where the thyroid gland produces an excessive amount of thyroid hormones. This is followed by a phase of hypothyroidism, where the thyroid gland fails to produce sufficient thyroid hormones. In some cases, the condition may resolve on its own, while others may experience long, term thyroid dysfunction.

Postpartum Graves' Disease:

Postpartum Graves' disease is a rare but serious condition characterized by an overactive thyroid gland. It is an autoimmune disorder in which the body's immune system mistakenly attacks the thyroid gland, causing it to produce excessive amounts of thyroid hormones. This can lead to symptoms such as weight loss, rapid heartbeat, anxiety, and tremors. Prompt medical intervention is crucial to manage this condition and prevent potential complications.

Impact on Postpartum Recovery:

Thyroid dysfunction can have a significant impact on postpartum recovery and overall well, being. The symptoms associated with both hyperthyroidism and hypothyroidism can interfere with a mother's ability to care for her newborn and adjust to her new role. Fatigue, weight fluctuations, mood changes, and difficulty concentrating can make the postpartum period challenging and overwhelming. Therefore, it is essential to recognize the signs and seek appropriate medical care to support a healthy recovery.

Management and Treatment:

Medical Evaluation:

If a woman experiences symptoms such as fatigue, mood swings, weight changes, or other signs of thyroid dysfunction, it is important to consult with a healthcare professional. A thorough medical evaluation, including a physical examination and blood tests to assess thyroid function, can help determine the appropriate course of action.

Medication:

Depending on the specific thyroid condition, medication may be prescribed to regulate thyroid hormone levels. In cases of hyperthyroidism, medications that block the production or release of thyroid hormones may be prescribed. For hypothyroidism, synthetic thyroid hormone replacement therapy may be necessary to restore normal thyroid function. It is important to take medication as prescribed and follow up with healthcare providers for regular monitoring.

Supportive Measures:

In addition to medical treatment, certain lifestyle adjustments can support postpartum recovery in the presence of thyroid dysfunction. These include:

Adequate rest and sleep: Prioritizing sleep and establishing a healthy sleep routine can help manage fatigue and promote overall well, being.

Balanced nutrition: Consuming a well, balanced diet that includes foods rich in iodine, selenium, and other essential nutrients can support thyroid function.

Stress management: Implementing stress, reduction techniques such as mindfulness, meditation, and gentle exercise can help alleviate symptoms and promote emotional well, being.

Recognizing the Symptoms

The postpartum period is a time of significant physical and emotional changes for new mothers. It is a period of recovery and adjustment as the body returns to its pre, pregnancy state. While each woman's postpartum experience is unique, it is essential to be aware of the common symptoms that may arise during this time. Recognizing these symptoms can help women seek appropriate support and take steps towards a healthy and smooth recovery. Below we will explore various aspects of postpartum recovery and discuss the importance of recognizing the symptoms associated with this transitional phase.

Physical Symptoms:

Pain and Discomfort:

Postpartum pain and discomfort are common as the body heals from childbirth. This can include pain at the site of a vaginal tear or episiotomy, soreness in the perineal area, and abdominal pain due to uterine contractions. It is important to manage pain with appropriate pain relief measures recommended by healthcare providers.

Vaginal Bleeding:

Postpartum bleeding, known as lochia, is a normal occurrence after childbirth. It typically lasts for a few weeks and gradually decreases in flow. However, if bleeding becomes excessively heavy, has a foul odor, or is accompanied by severe pain, it may indicate a complication and requires medical attention.

Breast Changes:

Breast engorgement, tenderness, and swelling are common as the body adjusts to breastfeeding. It is important to monitor for signs of mastitis, such as redness, fever, or flu, like symptoms, which may require medical intervention.

Urinary and Bowel Changes:

Postpartum women may experience changes in urinary and bowel habits. This can include increased frequency or urgency to urinate, difficulty initiating urination, or constipation. These changes are usually temporary but should be addressed if they persist or cause significant discomfort.

Emotional Symptoms:

Baby Blues:

The baby blues are a common phenomenon that occurs in the first week or two after childbirth. Women may experience mood swings, tearfulness, irritability, and feelings of sadness or anxiety. These symptoms are typically mild and resolve on their own. However, if they persist beyond two weeks or become more severe, it may be a sign of postpartum depression.

Postpartum Depression:

Postpartum depression is a more serious condition that can occur within the first year after childbirth. It involves persistent feelings of sadness, hopelessness, loss of interest in activities, changes in appetite and sleep patterns, difficulty bonding with the baby, and thoughts of self, harm or harm to the baby. It is crucial to recognize these symptoms and seek help from healthcare professionals to initiate appropriate treatment.

Postpartum Anxiety:

Postpartum anxiety is characterized by excessive worry, restlessness, racing thoughts, and physical symptoms such as heart palpitations or shortness of breath. It can coexist with or independently of postpartum depression. Seeking support from healthcare providers and mental health professionals is essential for managing postpartum anxiety.

Postpartum Psychosis:

Postpartum psychosis is a rare but severe condition that requires immediate medical attention. Symptoms include confusion, hallucinations, delusions, extreme agitation, and thoughts of harming oneself or the baby. This condition is considered a psychiatric emergency, and urgent intervention is necessary.

Seeking Support and Treatment:

Recognizing the symptoms of postpartum recovery is crucial, as it allows women to seek appropriate support and treatment. It is important for new mothers to reach out to their healthcare providers, family, and friends for assistance during this time. Support can come in various forms, including:

Seeking Proper Medical Care

The postpartum period is a critical phase in a woman's life, characterized by significant physical and emotional changes. It is essential for women to receive proper medical care during this time to ensure a healthy recovery and address any potential complications. Below we will explore the importance of seeking proper medical care in postpartum recovery, focusing on the various aspects of care that contribute to a woman's well, being.

Physical Health Monitoring:

After childbirth, a woman's body undergoes numerous changes as it returns to its pre, pregnancy state. Seeking proper medical care enables healthcare professionals to monitor and address any physical health concerns. Regular check, ups allow healthcare providers to assess vital signs, monitor healing progress, and address any postpartum complications. This includes monitoring blood pressure, checking incisions for signs of infection, and evaluating the overall healing process.

Additionally, medical care involves monitoring and supporting the reproductive organs' recovery, such as the uterus returning to its normal size and addressing any issues related to breastfeeding, urinary incontinence, or bowel movements. Regular visits to healthcare providers allow for early detection and intervention for any potential complications, promoting a healthy recovery.

Emotional and Mental Well, being:

Postpartum recovery involves not only physical healing but also emotional and mental well, being. The hormonal shifts, sleep deprivation, and adjustment to new responsibilities can contribute to mood changes and emotional challenges. Seeking proper medical care ensures that women receive the support they need for their emotional well, being.

Healthcare providers can screen for postpartum mood disorders, such as postpartum depression or anxiety, and provide appropriate interventions. They can offer guidance on self, care strategies, coping mechanisms, and referrals to mental health professionals if necessary. Open communication with healthcare providers allows women to discuss their emotional well, being, seek help when needed, and receive the necessary support to navigate this vulnerable period.

Education and Guidance:

Proper medical care during the postpartum period provides women with essential education and guidance. Healthcare providers can offer information on postpartum recovery, including what to expect physically and emotionally, common discomforts, and warning signs to watch out for. This knowledge empowers women to understand their bodies and make informed decisions regarding their recovery.

Healthcare professionals can also provide guidance on nutrition, exercise, and self, care practices that support postpartum healing. This includes recommendations on a balanced diet to promote healing, appropriate exercises to regain strength, and strategies to manage fatigue and stress. Access to accurate and reliable information through medical care equips women with the tools and knowledge necessary for a successful postpartum recovery.

Breastfeeding Support:

For women who choose to breastfeed, proper medical care is vital to ensure successful lactation and address any breastfeeding challenges. Healthcare providers can offer guidance on establishing proper latch, managing engorgement or nipple soreness, and ensuring an adequate milk supply. They can also assess infant growth and provide resources for additional lactation support if needed.

Furthermore, medical care can address any medical conditions that may impact breastfeeding, such as breast infections or mastitis. Timely intervention and support from healthcare providers enhance the breastfeeding experience and contribute to both the mother's and the baby's overall well, being.

Continuity of Care:

Seeking proper medical care in the postpartum period establishes a foundation for ongoing healthcare and wellness. Regular check, ups and communication with healthcare providers create a continuity of care that extends beyond the immediate postpartum phase. It allows for the ongoing management of chronic conditions, such as hypertension or diabetes, and promotes overall health and wellness in the long term.

Additionally, continuity of care ensures that women have access to contraceptive counseling and family planning services, enabling them to make informed decisions about their reproductive health and future pregnancies.

Chapter Twenty-Two

Birth Control After Baby

The postpartum period is a time of physical and emotional recovery for women after childbirth. It is also an important time to consider and discuss birth control options. Birth control not only helps prevent unwanted pregnancies but also plays a crucial role in a woman's overall well, being and family planning. Below we will explore the various birth control options available to women after childbirth and their relevance in the context of postpartum recovery.

The Importance of Birth Control in Postpartum Recovery:

Understanding the importance of birth control in the postpartum period is essential. After giving birth, a woman's body needs time to heal and recover. It is recommended to wait at least six weeks before resuming sexual activity to allow the body to heal adequately. However, this does not eliminate the risk of pregnancy, as ovulation can occur before the return of menstrual periods. Therefore, discussing and implementing a reliable method of birth control is crucial to prevent unintended pregnancies and promote postpartum recovery.

Barrier Methods:

Barrier methods of birth control offer convenience and effectiveness, especially in the postpartum period. Options such as condoms or diaphragms provide a physical barrier that prevents sperm from reaching the egg. They are easily accessible, have minimal side effects, and can be used immediately after childbirth. However, it is important to ensure proper usage and adherence to maximize their effectiveness.

Hormonal Methods:

Hormonal methods of birth control are widely used and highly effective. They work by preventing ovulation and altering the cervical mucus to inhibit sperm movement. Several hormonal options are available to women postpartum, including:

Combination Oral Contraceptives: These pills contain synthetic versions of estrogen and progestin hormones. While they are effective and offer non, contraceptive benefits such as regulating menstrual cycles and reducing menstrual pain, they may not be recommended immediately after childbirth due to the potential impact on breastfeeding.

Progestin, Only Pills: Also known as mini, pills, these pills contain only progestin hormone. They are considered safe for breastfeeding mothers and can be initiated soon after childbirth. They require strict adherence to a specific daily schedule to ensure effectiveness.

Progestin, Only Injections: Injections such as Depo, Provera provide three months of contraception with a single shot. They offer convenience for women who may have difficulty remembering to take pills regularly. However, it is important to note that they may cause a temporary delay in fertility after discontinuation.

Progestin, Only Implants: Implants like Nexplanon are small, flexible rods placed under the skin of the upper arm. They provide long, term contraception for up to three years, making them a convenient option for postpartum women. They are safe for breastfeeding mothers and have a high efficacy rate.

Intrauterine Devices (IUDs):

IUDs are a popular and effective form of long, acting reversible contraception. They are inserted into the uterus by a healthcare provider and can provide protection against pregnancy for several years. There are two types of IUDs available:

Copper IUD: This non, hormonal option works by creating an environment toxic to sperm, preventing fertilization. Copper IUDs are safe for breastfeeding mothers and can provide contraception for up to ten years.

Hormonal IUD: These IUDs release a low dose of progestin hormone into the uterus, thinning the uterine lining and thickening cervical mucus. They are safe for breastfeeding mothers and can provide contraception for three to five years, depending on the brand.

IUDs are reversible and can be removed at any time, allowing for quick return to fertility once removed.

Understanding Your Options

The postpartum period is a transformative time for women, both physically and emotionally. It is crucial for new mothers to understand their options and make informed decisions regarding their postpartum recovery. Below we will explore various aspects of postpartum recovery and the options available to women during this time. By understanding and exploring these options, women can make choices that promote their overall well, being and enhance their postpartum recovery journey.

Physical Recovery:

Physical recovery is an essential aspect of postpartum well, being. The body goes through significant changes during pregnancy and childbirth, and allowing ample time for recovery is crucial. Some key aspects of physical recovery include:

Rest and Sleep: Adequate rest and sleep are vital for the body to heal and recover. It is important for new mothers to prioritize sleep, nap when the baby sleeps, and seek support from partners, family members, or friends to ensure sufficient rest.

Nutrition: Proper nutrition is essential for postpartum recovery. A balanced diet rich in nutrients can promote healing, provide energy, and support breastfeeding. Women should focus on consuming a variety of fruits, vegetables, lean proteins, whole grains, and healthy fats.

Exercise: Engaging in gentle exercises and postpartum, specific workouts can help restore muscle strength, improve cardiovascular health, and enhance overall well, being. It is important to consult with healthcare professionals before starting any exercise regimen.

Emotional Well, being:

Emotional well, being plays a significant role in postpartum recovery. Hormonal changes, sleep deprivation, and the demands of caring for a newborn can impact a woman's mental health. It is important to prioritize emotional well, being and seek support when needed. Some strategies for supporting emotional well, being include:

Open Communication: Talking openly about feelings and experiences with loved ones, friends, or healthcare professionals can provide emotional support and validation.

Self, care: Engaging in self, care activities, such as taking a warm bath, practicing mindfulness or meditation, pursuing hobbies, or seeking relaxation techniques, can help reduce stress and promote emotional well, being.

Support Networks: Building a support network of friends, family, or joining postpartum support groups can provide a sense of community and facilitate sharing experiences with other mothers.

Bonding with Your Baby:

Bonding with your baby is a vital aspect of postpartum recovery. Developing a strong bond promotes emotional well, being for both the mother and the baby. Some strategies to enhance bonding include:

Skin, to, skin Contact: Engaging in skin, to, skin contact with the baby promotes bonding, regulates the baby's body temperature, and facilitates breastfeeding.

Breastfeeding: Breastfeeding provides an opportunity for close physical contact and releases hormones that promote maternal, infant bonding.

Baby Massage: Gentle baby massage techniques can promote relaxation, improve circulation, and enhance the bond between mother and baby.

Postpartum Support:

Seeking postpartum support can significantly contribute to a woman's recovery journey. It is important to know the resources available and reach out for support when needed. Some postpartum support options include:

1Postpartum Doula: A postpartum doula provides practical support, guidance, and assistance to new mothers during the postpartum period. They can help with newborn care, household tasks, and provide emotional support.

1Support Groups: Joining postpartum support groups or online communities can offer a sense of connection and provide a space for sharing experiences, concerns, and advice.

Healthcare Professionals: Regular check, ups with healthcare professionals allow for monitoring of physical and emotional well, being. They can provide guidance on recovery, address concerns, and offer resources for support.

Discussing Birth Control with Your Doctor

The postpartum period is a significant phase in a woman's life, marked by physical and emotional changes as well as the joy of welcoming a new baby. During this time, it is important for women to consider their contraceptive options to prevent unintended pregnancies and support their postpartum recovery. Below we will explore the importance of discussing birth control with your healthcare provider in the context of postpartum recovery. Understanding and evaluating birth control options can empower women to make informed decisions that align with their reproductive goals and overall well, being.

The Importance of Postpartum Birth Control:

After giving birth, many women may not be ready for another pregnancy right away. It is crucial to understand that fertility can return soon after childbirth, even if breastfeeding. Thus, discussing birth control with a healthcare provider is essential to ensure effective contraception and support the mother's physical and emotional recovery. Key reasons to consider postpartum birth control include:

Preventing Unintended Pregnancies: Contraception allows women to plan their pregnancies and ensure that they are physically, emotionally, and financially prepared for another child.

Supporting Physical Recovery: Adequate spacing between pregnancies allows the body to heal, replenish nutritional stores, and recover from the demands of childbirth.

Emotional Well, being: Nurturing and bonding with a newborn requires emotional energy and attention. Birth control can provide women with the peace of mind to focus on their own recovery and their new baby without the added stress of a potential unintended pregnancy.

Discussing Birth Control Options:

When discussing birth control with your healthcare provider, it is important to consider various factors, including:

Timing: The choice of birth control may depend on whether a woman is breastfeeding or has resumed menstruation. Some contraceptive methods may have an impact on milk supply or be more suitable after the return of regular menstrual cycles.

Effectiveness: Understanding the effectiveness rates of different contraceptive methods is important for making an informed decision. Options range from hormonal methods like the pill, patch, or IUDs, to barrier methods like condoms, or long, acting reversible contraceptives (LARC) such as the implant or intrauterine devices.

Side Effects: Discussing potential side effects of birth control methods is essential to find an option that aligns with a woman's overall health and well, being. It is important to note that some hormonal methods may have different effects on breastfeeding, mood, or menstrual cycles.

Contraceptive Counseling: Healthcare providers play a crucial role in providing information, guidance, and counseling regarding contraceptive options. They can discuss the pros and cons of different methods, address concerns, and help women choose the most suitable option based on their individual needs and preferences.

Postpartum Recovery Considerations:

During the postpartum period, women may have specific considerations when choosing a birth control method. These considerations include:

Breastfeeding: If a woman is breastfeeding, she may prefer non, hormonal or progestin, only contraceptive methods to minimize potential impacts on milk supply.

Hormonal Changes: The postpartum period is characterized by fluctuating hormone levels. Some women may experience irregular periods or hormonal imbalances, which can be considered when discussing hormonal contraceptive options.

1Future Family Planning: Women's reproductive goals and plans may also influence their choice of birth control. Some methods are reversible and allow for prompt return of fertility, while others provide longer, term protection.

Communication and Follow, up:

Effective communication with healthcare providers is crucial throughout the postpartum period. It is important to:

1Be Open and Honest: Share your preferences, concerns, and any relevant medical history with your healthcare provider. This will help them understand your needs and provide appropriate guidance.

Chapter Twenty-Three

Postpartum Sleep

The postpartum period is a transformative time for new mothers, marked by joy, love, and the challenges of caring for a newborn. During this phase, it is essential for women to prioritize their physical and mental well, being, and one key aspect of that is getting adequate sleep. Below we will explore the importance of sleep in postpartum recovery and discuss strategies to promote better sleep quality for new mothers.

The Sleep Challenges of Postpartum Period:

The arrival of a newborn can significantly disrupt a mother's sleep patterns. The following factors contribute to the sleep challenges experienced by postpartum women:

Frequent Nighttime Feedings: Newborns have small stomachs and need to eat frequently, leading to interrupted sleep for mothers who need to attend to their baby's feeding needs throughout the night.

Irregular Sleep Patterns: Newborns do not follow a predictable sleep, wake cycle, making it challenging for mothers to establish a regular sleep routine.

Discomfort and Pain: Postpartum physical changes, such as perineal soreness or C, section incisions, can cause discomfort and pain, making it harder for women to find a comfortable sleeping position.

Hormonal Changes: Fluctuating hormone levels, including the decrease in estrogen and progesterone after childbirth, can affect sleep patterns and quality.

The Importance of Sleep in Postpartum Recovery:

Adequate sleep plays a crucial role in postpartum recovery and overall well, being. Here are some reasons why sleep is important during this period:

Physical Healing: Sleep promotes the body's healing process, allowing tissues to repair, hormones to rebalance, and energy levels to replenish. Quality sleep can help new mothers recover from the physical demands of childbirth.

Mental Health and Emotional Well, being: Sleep deprivation can have a significant impact on mental health, increasing the risk of postpartum depression and anxiety. Getting enough sleep allows for better emotional regulation, mood stability, and overall mental well, being.

Cognitive Function: Sleep is essential for cognitive processes, including memory consolidation, attention, and decision, making. Adequate sleep can help new mothers stay alert and focused during their daily tasks, including caring for their baby.

Energy and Stamina: The demands of caring for a newborn require energy and stamina. Sufficient sleep helps replenish energy levels, enabling mothers to tackle the challenges of motherhood with greater resilience.

Strategies for Better Sleep in the Postpartum Period:

Although it can be challenging to achieve uninterrupted sleep with a newborn, there are strategies that can promote better sleep quality and recovery during the postpartum period:

Sleep When the Baby Sleeps: New mothers should prioritize rest and take advantage of their baby's sleep periods to nap and recharge. This can help compensate for the lack of consolidated sleep during the night.

Establish a Bedtime Routine: Creating a relaxing bedtime routine can signal to the body that it's time to wind down and prepare for sleep. Activities such as taking a warm bath, reading a book, or practicing relaxation techniques can help promote better sleep onset.

1Share Nighttime Responsibilities: If possible, share nighttime responsibilities with a partner or other supportive family members. Taking turns caring for the baby during the night can ensure that both parents have an opportunity to get adequate rest.

1Optimize Sleep Environment: Create a sleep, friendly environment by keeping the bedroom cool, dark, and quiet. Consider using earplugs, an eye mask, or a white noise machine to drown out external noises and promote uninterrupted sleep.

Seek Support: Reach out to family members, friends, or postpartum support groups for assistance and support. Having someone to talk to and share the challenges of sleep deprivation can alleviate some of the emotional and mental strain.

The Impact of Sleep Deprivation

The postpartum period is a time of immense joy and adjustment as new mothers navigate the challenges of caring for their newborns. During this phase, sleep deprivation can have a profound impact on a mother's physical and mental well, being, as well as her ability to recover from childbirth. Below we will explore the effects of sleep deprivation on postpartum recovery and discuss strategies to address this issue.

Sleep Deprivation and Physical Recovery:

Sleep deprivation can hinder the body's ability to heal and recover from the physical demands of childbirth. Here are some ways sleep deprivation can impact postpartum physical recovery:

Impaired Wound Healing: Sleep is crucial for the body's natural healing processes. Lack of sleep can delay wound healing, such as perineal tears or C, section incisions, increasing the risk of complications and prolonging recovery time.

Decreased Immune Function: Sleep deprivation weakens the immune system, leaving new mothers vulnerable to infections and illnesses. A compromised immune system can slow down the healing process and prolong postpartum recovery.

Increased Pain Sensitivity: Sleep deprivation can heighten pain sensitivity. New mothers who are sleep, deprived may experience increased pain perception, making postpartum discomfort and physical recovery more challenging.

Hormonal Imbalances: Sleep deprivation disrupts hormonal balance, including the production of growth hormone and prolactin, which are essential for tissue repair and breastfeeding. Hormonal imbalances can further hinder the body's ability to recover after childbirth.

Sleep Deprivation and Mental Health:

Sleep deprivation can have a significant impact on a new mother's mental health and emotional well, being. The postpartum period already poses unique emotional challenges, and sleep deprivation exacerbates these issues. Here's how sleep deprivation affects mental health:

Increased Risk of Postpartum Depression: Sleep deprivation is closely linked to an increased risk of postpartum depression. The hormonal and emotional changes during the postpartum period, combined with a lack of sleep, can contribute to the development of depression and anxiety disorders.

Emotional Instability: Sleep deprivation impairs emotional regulation, making new mothers more prone to mood swings, irritability, and feelings of overwhelm. This emotional instability can interfere with the bonding process and overall well, being.

Impaired Cognitive Function: Lack of sleep affects cognitive function, including memory, concentration, and decision, making abilities. Sleep, deprived new mothers may struggle to focus, make decisions, and perform daily tasks effectively.

Strategies for Addressing Sleep Deprivation:

Recognizing the importance of adequate sleep in postpartum recovery, here are some strategies to help new mothers combat sleep deprivation and promote better sleep:

Establish a Sleep Routine: Creating a consistent bedtime routine can signal to the body that it's time to sleep. Engage in relaxing activities before bed, such as taking a warm bath, reading a book, or practicing relaxation techniques.

Take Naps: Napping during the day can help compensate for the interrupted sleep at night. Whenever the baby sleeps, new mothers should prioritize rest and take short naps to recharge.

Seek Support: Reach out to partners, family members, or friends for support. Having someone to share nighttime responsibilities can ensure that new mothers have the opportunity to get uninterrupted sleep.

1Create a Restful Environment: Make the sleep environment conducive to relaxation and rest. Keep the bedroom cool, dark, and quiet. Use blackout curtains, earplugs, or a white noise machine to block out disturbances.

1Practice Sleep Hygiene: Adopt healthy sleep habits, such as avoiding stimulants like caffeine and electronic devices before bed. Maintain a consistent sleep, wake schedule, even on weekends, to regulate the body's internal clock.

Tips for Better Sleep

The postpartum period is a transformative and joyous time for new mothers, but it can also be physically and emotionally demanding. One of the biggest challenges during this phase is getting enough sleep. Sleep plays a crucial role in postpartum recovery, aiding in physical healing, emotional well, being, and overall adjustment to motherhood. Below we will explore various tips for better sleep during the postpartum period and their relevance to the recovery process.

Prioritize Sleep:

Recognize that sleep is essential for your well, being and recovery. Prioritize sleep as a top priority and make it a non, negotiable part of your daily routine. Aim to get as much sleep as possible, especially during the early postpartum weeks when your body needs ample rest to heal.

Sleep When the Baby Sleeps:

One of the most common pieces of advice given to new mothers is to sleep when the baby sleeps. It's essential to take advantage of these opportunities to rest and recharge. By aligning your sleep schedule with your baby's sleep patterns, you can maximize your rest time and reduce sleep deprivation.

Establish a Bedtime Routine:

Creating a consistent bedtime routine can signal to your body that it's time to wind down and prepare for sleep. Develop a relaxing routine that suits your preferences and helps you transition from the demands of the day to a more peaceful state. This could include activities like taking a warm bath, reading a book, practicing deep breathing exercises, or listening to soothing music.

Create a Sleep, Conducive Environment:

Make your sleep environment as comfortable and conducive to rest as possible. Keep your bedroom cool, dark, and quiet. Invest in comfortable bedding and a supportive mattress. Use blackout curtains or an eye mask to block out any unwanted light. Consider using earplugs or a white noise machine to drown out noise disturbances that may disrupt your sleep.

Seek Support:

Don't hesitate to seek support from your partner, family members, or friends. Let them know that you need help with nighttime feedings or other responsibilities so that you can get uninterrupted sleep. Having a support system in place can alleviate some of the stress and allow you to focus on prioritizing your sleep.

Practice Healthy Sleep Hygiene:

Adopting good sleep hygiene practices can significantly improve your sleep quality. Here are some recommendations:

Avoid consuming caffeine and other stimulants close to bedtime as they can interfere with your ability to fall asleep.

Establish a regular sleep schedule by going to bed and waking up at consistent times each day.

Create a relaxing pre, sleep routine that helps you unwind and signals to your body that it's time to sleep.

Limit exposure to electronic devices, such as smartphones and tablets, before bed as the blue light emitted can disrupt your sleep, wake cycle.

Ensure your bedroom is a peaceful and comfortable environment, free from distractions.

Practice Stress Management Techniques:

Stress and anxiety can make it difficult to fall asleep and stay asleep. Engage in stress management techniques to help calm your mind and promote relaxation. This can include activities such as meditation, deep breathing exercises, gentle yoga, or journaling. Find what works best for you and incorporate it into your daily routine.

Consider Co, Sleeping or Room, Sharing:

If you're comfortable with the idea and follow safety guidelines, co, sleeping or room, sharing with your baby can make nighttime feedings and comforting more convenient. Being close to your baby can help you respond quickly to their needs, allowing you to settle back to sleep more easily afterward.

Take Power Naps:

During the day, if you're feeling particularly tired or sleep, deprived, taking power naps can provide a quick boost of energy.

Chapter Twenty-Four

The Second Baby: What's Different?

Welcoming a second baby into the family is an exciting and unique experience. While some aspects of caring for a newborn may feel familiar from your previous parenting journey, there are also differences that come with having a second child. Below we will explore the various factors that make the arrival of a second baby distinct from the first, particularly in relation to postpartum recovery. We'll delve into the physical, emotional, and logistical aspects of this transition and provide valuable insights for parents navigating this new chapter.

Physical Changes and Recovery:

One significant difference between the first and second baby is the physical changes and recovery process. While the body goes through similar changes during pregnancy and childbirth, the recovery may vary depending on the birth experience and the mother's overall health. It's important to give yourself ample time to heal, even if you have experience with postpartum recovery. Your body may have different needs and challenges this time around. Engaging in self, care practices, such as getting adequate rest, eating nutritious meals, and seeking support, will help facilitate a smoother recovery.

Emotional Adjustment:

Emotionally, the arrival of a second baby brings about a unique set of feelings. While the bond with your first child is already established, the challenge lies in finding a balance between meeting the needs of both children and ensuring that your firstborn feels loved and supported during this transition. It's normal to experience a range of emotions, including joy, excitement, and even feelings of guilt or apprehension. Taking time for self, reflection and seeking emotional support can be beneficial in navigating these complex emotions.

Logistical Considerations:

When it comes to logistics, having a second baby introduces new considerations. For instance, adjusting to the demands of caring for multiple children can be challenging, especially in the early days when sleep deprivation and round, the, clock care are essential. Finding a routine that works for the entire family can help streamline daily activities and ease the adjustment period. Additionally, managing the responsibilities of a growing family may require delegating tasks, seeking help from family or friends, or exploring childcare options that suit your needs.

Sibling Dynamics and Relationships:

One significant aspect of having a second baby is the impact it has on sibling dynamics and relationships. Your firstborn may experience a range of emotions, from excitement and curiosity to jealousy and insecurity. It's important to foster a supportive environment where both children feel loved and included. Encouraging sibling bonding, involving the older child in caring for the baby, and setting aside special one, on, one time with each child can help nurture positive sibling relationships and mitigate any potential feelings of rivalry or resentment.

Postpartum Support and Resources:

Seeking postpartum support and utilizing available resources becomes even more crucial with a second baby. Postpartum support can come in various forms, such as enlisting the help of family and friends, hiring a postpartum doula, or joining support groups specifically designed for parents with multiple children. These resources provide valuable guidance, encouragement, and a sense of community, which can contribute to a smoother postpartum recovery and adjustment period.

Managing Time and Self, Care:

Time management and self, care become increasingly important when caring for multiple children. It's vital to carve out moments for self, care, even in the midst of a busy schedule. Prioritizing self, care activities, such as exercise, rest, engaging in hobbies, and maintaining social connections, helps to recharge and nurture your well, being. Remember that taking care of yourself allows you to be fully present and available for your children's needs.

Balancing Parental Attention:

Finding a balance between attending to the needs of both children can be a juggling act. Each child requires individual attention, and as parents, it's important to allocate time and resources accordingly.

Preparing for Another Pregnancy

Welcoming another pregnancy into your life is an exciting and transformative experience. Whether you're planning to expand your family soon after your previous pregnancy or taking some time before embarking on the journey again, proper preparation is key. Below we will explore the importance of preparing for another pregnancy, particularly in relation to postpartum recovery. We'll discuss various factors to consider, including physical and emotional health, lifestyle adjustments, and medical guidance, to ensure a smooth and healthy transition into this next phase of parenthood.

Physical Health and Well, being:

One of the essential aspects of preparing for another pregnancy is focusing on physical health and well, being. Before conceiving, it's crucial to optimize your overall health by maintaining a balanced diet, engaging in regular exercise, and getting regular check, ups with your healthcare provider. Adequate nutrition and regular physical activity not only support your own well, being but also create an optimal environment for the development of a healthy baby. Additionally, addressing any pre, existing health conditions and ensuring they are properly managed is vital in ensuring a successful pregnancy and postpartum recovery.

Postpartum Recovery:

Considering the postpartum recovery period is an integral part of preparing for another pregnancy. Reflecting on your previous postpartum experience and identifying any areas that could be improved will help you better prepare for the next recovery period. If you encountered challenges during your previous postpartum journey, it's important to address them and seek appropriate support or resources. This might include consulting with a healthcare provider, joining postpartum support groups, or seeking the assistance of a postpartum doula. By proactively addressing postpartum recovery, you can create a more positive and supported experience for yourself and your baby.

Emotional Well, being:

Preparing for another pregnancy also involves addressing your emotional well, being. Pregnancy and the postpartum period can bring about a range of emotions, and it's important to be in a stable and supportive emotional state before embarking on another pregnancy journey. Reflect on your emotional experiences during your previous pregnancy and postpartum period. Consider whether you would benefit from therapy or counseling to address any unresolved emotional issues. Seeking emotional support and engaging in self, care practices, such as mindfulness, relaxation techniques, and maintaining social connections, will contribute to your overall emotional well, being during this time.

Lifestyle Adjustments:

Another aspect of preparing for another pregnancy is making necessary lifestyle adjustments. This might include reassessing your work, life balance, adjusting your exercise routine, and making modifications to your daily routine to accommodate the needs of a growing family. Consider how you can create a supportive and nurturing environment for yourself and your future baby. This may involve delegating tasks, enlisting the help of family and friends, or exploring childcare options. By proactively addressing these lifestyle adjustments, you can better manage your responsibilities and create a harmonious balance between your personal life and the demands of pregnancy and motherhood.

Medical Guidance and Preconception Care:

Seeking medical guidance and preconception care is vital when preparing for another pregnancy. Schedule a preconception appointment with your healthcare provider to discuss your plans and receive personalized advice based on your medical history and specific needs. This appointment will allow your healthcare provider to assess your overall health, review any potential risks or concerns, and provide recommendations for optimizing your chances of a healthy pregnancy. Additionally, your healthcare provider may discuss prenatal vitamins, recommended screenings or tests, and any necessary vaccinations to ensure a safe and healthy pregnancy journey.

Addressing Infertility or Pregnancy Loss:

If you've experienced infertility or pregnancy loss in the past, preparing for another pregnancy may involve additional considerations. Consult with a fertility specialist or reproductive endocrinologist to discuss your options and develop a comprehensive plan that addresses any underlying fertility issues or concerns.

Recovery Differences with Subsequent Children

The journey of postpartum recovery is a unique experience for every new mother. It is a period of physical and emotional healing as well as adjustment to the demands of caring for a newborn. While each postpartum recovery is significant, it's important to recognize that subsequent pregnancies and births may bring about different recovery experiences. Below we will explore the recovery differences that women may encounter with subsequent children, shedding light on the factors that contribute to these variations. Understanding these differences can empower women to navigate their postpartum recovery with knowledge and support.

Physical Recovery:

Physical recovery after childbirth can vary with subsequent pregnancies. Women who have previously given birth may find that their bodies recover more quickly, as their muscles and tissues have gone through the process of pregnancy and childbirth before. However, the physical recovery can still be influenced by factors such as the spacing between pregnancies, the mode of delivery, and the overall health of the mother.

Spacing between pregnancies: The spacing between pregnancies can play a role in the physical recovery. A shorter gap between pregnancies may pose additional challenges to the body's ability to fully recover. The body may not have had enough time to regain its strength and heal before the demands of another pregnancy and childbirth occur. On the other hand, a longer gap between pregnancies allows for more time for the body to recover, leading to a potentially smoother postpartum experience.

Mode of delivery: The mode of delivery also impacts the physical recovery with subsequent children. Women who have previously had a vaginal birth may find that their bodies are better prepared for subsequent vaginal deliveries. However, if a previous birth was a cesarean section, the recovery from subsequent c, sections may involve additional considerations. The healing of the incision site and the recovery of abdominal muscles can take longer compared to vaginal births. It is essential for women to follow their healthcare provider's advice on postoperative care and engage in appropriate exercises to strengthen the abdominal muscles.

Overall health: The overall health of the mother can significantly influence the physical recovery. A healthy lifestyle, including regular exercise, a nutritious diet, and adequate rest, can contribute to a smoother recovery. Prioritizing self, care and listening to one's body's needs are essential in supporting physical healing and well, being. Additionally, addressing any pre, existing health conditions and seeking appropriate medical care will positively impact the recovery process.

Emotional Well, being:

Emotional well, being is another aspect of postpartum recovery that can vary with subsequent children. While some women may feel more confident and emotionally prepared for the challenges of motherhood after having previous children, others may experience new emotional dynamics and adjustments. Factors such as the demands of caring for multiple children, different personalities and needs of each child, and changes in family dynamics can influence emotional well, being.

Caring for multiple children: Caring for multiple children can bring added responsibilities and challenges. Juggling the needs of multiple children, managing schedules, and finding a balance between individual attention and collective care can be emotionally demanding. Women may experience feelings of overwhelm or guilt as they navigate the complexities of meeting the needs of each child. Building a support network, seeking help from family and friends, and practicing self, care become even more important during this time.

Individual needs and personalities: Each child has unique needs and personalities, which can impact a mother's emotional well, being. Women may find that the challenges they faced with their previous children do not necessarily apply to subsequent children. It's essential to adapt parenting strategies and find what works best for each child. This flexibility and acceptance of individual differences can alleviate stress and support a positive emotional experience.

Chapter Twenty-Five

Building a Postpartum Support Network

The postpartum period is a time of immense change and transition for new mothers. It is a time of physical recovery, emotional adjustment, and the steep learning curve of caring for a newborn. While this journey can be beautiful and rewarding, it can also be challenging and overwhelming. Therefore, having a strong support network is essential to ensure a smooth postpartum recovery. Below we will explore the importance of building a postpartum support network, the benefits it provides, and practical steps to create a network that promotes postpartum well, being.

Understanding the Importance of a Postpartum Support Network:

A postpartum support network consists of individuals who provide emotional, physical, and practical support during the postpartum period. This network plays a crucial role in facilitating the recovery process and promoting the overall well, being of new mothers. Here are some key reasons why building a postpartum support network is essential:

Emotional Support: The postpartum period can bring a range of emotions, including joy, exhaustion, anxiety, and even feelings of isolation. Having a support network allows new mothers to share their experiences, concerns, and emotions with trusted individuals who can provide empathy, understanding, and encouragement. This emotional support can help alleviate stress, reduce feelings of loneliness, and promote mental well, being.

Practical Assistance: Caring for a newborn is a demanding task that requires physical stamina and constant attention. A support network can offer practical assistance, such as helping with household chores, preparing meals, or providing childcare for older siblings. This practical support allows new mothers to focus on their own recovery and bonding with their baby without feeling overwhelmed by the daily tasks of running a household.

Knowledge and Information: Building a support network provides access to a wealth of knowledge and experience. Trusted individuals within the network, such as experienced mothers, healthcare professionals, or lactation consultants, can offer valuable advice and guidance on various aspects of postpartum recovery. This information can empower new mothers to make informed decisions about their own health, the care of their newborn, and navigate any challenges that may arise.

Sense of Community: Feeling connected to others who are going through or have gone through a similar experience can be immensely comforting. Being part of a support network allows new mothers to share their joys and struggles, exchange stories, and find solace in knowing that they are not alone on their postpartum journey. This sense of community fosters a supportive and non, judgmental environment where new mothers can seek guidance, ask questions, and receive validation.

Building a Postpartum Support Network:

Creating a postpartum support network requires proactive effort and careful consideration. Here are some practical steps to build a strong support network:

Identify Key Individuals: Start by identifying the people in your life who can provide support during the postpartum period. This may include your partner, family members, close friends, and even neighbors or community members who have offered assistance. Consider their availability, reliability, and willingness to help during this crucial time.

Communicate Your Needs: Clearly communicate your needs and expectations to your support network. Express your desire for emotional support, practical assistance, or specific areas where you may need guidance. Open and honest communication will ensure that your support network understands how they can best support you.

Seek Professional Support: In addition to family and friends, professional support can be invaluable during the postpartum period. Consult with healthcare professionals, such as your obstetrician, midwife, or a postpartum doula. These professionals can provide specialized care, guidance, and resources tailored to your unique needs.

The Importance of Community

The postpartum period is a transformative and delicate phase in a woman's life. It is a time when mothers navigate physical recovery, emotional adjustments, and the responsibilities of caring for a newborn. During this vulnerable time, the support and connection offered by a community can make a significant difference in a mother's postpartum recovery. Below we will explore the importance of community in relation to postpartum recovery, the benefits it provides, and how it can positively impact a mother's well, being.

Building a Supportive Community:

A supportive community plays a vital role in the postpartum recovery journey. Here are some reasons why community support is essential:

Emotional Support: The postpartum period can bring a range of emotions, including joy, excitement, but also anxiety, fatigue, and mood swings. Having a community of understanding individuals can provide a safe space for mothers to express their feelings, fears, and challenges without judgment. Emotional support helps alleviate stress, reduces feelings of isolation, and promotes overall mental well, being.

Validation and Empathy: Connecting with others who have gone through or are going through similar experiences helps mothers feel validated and understood. Sharing stories, concerns, and triumphs with fellow mothers creates a sense of belonging and reassurance that they are not alone in their struggles. This shared empathy fosters a supportive environment where mothers can find comfort, advice, and encouragement.

Practical Assistance: The postpartum period comes with physical challenges and increased responsibilities. Having a community of friends, family members, or neighbors who are willing to lend a helping hand can make a significant difference. Practical support can include assistance with household chores, meal preparation, running errands, or even providing childcare, allowing the mother to prioritize self, care and focus on her recovery.

Access to Information and Resources: Being part of a community provides access to a wealth of knowledge and resources. Other mothers who have experienced postpartum recovery can share their insights, tips, and advice on various aspects of caring for a newborn, breastfeeding, sleep routines, and self, care practices. Additionally, community networks may connect mothers to healthcare professionals, lactation consultants, or support groups specializing in postpartum recovery.

Peer Learning and Growth: Engaging with a supportive community allows mothers to learn from one another's experiences, successes, and challenges. Sharing information, exchanging ideas, and seeking advice from trusted individuals in the community can broaden a mother's knowledge base and empower her to make informed decisions about her postpartum recovery journey.

Creating and Nurturing a Supportive Community:

Building a strong and supportive community requires proactive effort and intentional connections. Here are some practical ways to create and nurture a community during the postpartum period:

Engage in Prenatal Classes and Support Groups: Attending prenatal classes or support groups provides an opportunity to connect with other expectant mothers who are going through a similar journey. These groups often continue postpartum, allowing mothers to maintain relationships and find comfort in sharing their experiences.

Seek Online Communities: The internet offers a vast array of online communities and forums dedicated to postpartum recovery. Joining these platforms can connect mothers with individuals who understand their challenges and provide valuable support, advice, and information.

Connect with Local Parenting Organizations: Explore local parenting organizations, motherhood groups, or community centers that offer support and activities for new mothers. Participating in events, workshops, or mom, and, baby classes creates opportunities to connect with like, minded individuals.

Cultivate Relationships with Family and Friends: Strengthen existing relationships with family and friends by communicating your needs and expressing your desire for support during the postpartum period.

Finding Your Tribe

Finding Your Tribe: Building a Supportive Community for Postpartum Recovery

The postpartum period is a transformative and challenging time for new mothers. It is a time of physical healing, emotional adjustment, and navigating the responsibilities of caring for a newborn. During this phase, having a supportive community, often referred to as your "tribe," can make a significant difference in a mother's postpartum recovery. Below we will explore the importance of finding your tribe, the benefits it provides, and how it can positively impact a mother's well, being during the postpartum period.

Building a Supportive Tribe:

Finding your tribe involves surrounding yourself with individuals who provide support, understanding, and encouragement during the postpartum journey. Here are some key reasons why building a supportive tribe is crucial for postpartum recovery:

Emotional Support: The postpartum period can be emotionally overwhelming. Hormonal changes, sleep deprivation, and the challenges of adjusting to motherhood can lead to a rollercoaster of emotions. Having a tribe of understanding individuals who can listen, empathize, and offer guidance provides a safe space for expressing emotions without judgment. Emotional support from your tribe helps alleviate stress, reduces feelings of isolation, and promotes overall mental well, being.

Practical Assistance: Caring for a newborn requires significant physical and mental energy. Your tribe can provide practical assistance in the form of helping with household chores, meal preparation, or running errands.

They can also offer support by babysitting, allowing you to take breaks for self, care or rest. The practical assistance provided by your tribe lightens the load and enables you to focus on your postpartum recovery.

Validation and Understanding: Connecting with other mothers who have experienced or are currently going through the postpartum journey can provide a sense of validation and understanding. Sharing experiences, concerns, and triumphs with your tribe allows you to realize that you are not alone in your struggles. Your tribe can offer reassurance, advice, and a shoulder to lean on during challenging times.

Peer Learning and Growth: Building a tribe allows for peer learning and growth. Each member of your tribe brings unique experiences and perspectives, which can broaden your knowledge and understanding of postpartum recovery. Sharing information, exchanging tips, and seeking advice from trusted tribe members can empower you to make informed decisions about your recovery journey.

Finding Your Tribe:

Building a supportive tribe takes effort and intentionality. Here are some practical steps to help you find your tribe during the postpartum period:

Join Postpartum Support Groups: Look for local postpartum support groups in your community or online. These groups provide an opportunity to connect with other mothers who are going through a similar experience. Sharing your journey, asking questions, and receiving support from group members can be immensely beneficial.

Attend Mommy, and, Baby Classes: Participate in mommy, and, baby classes or activities in your area. These classes not only allow you to bond with your baby but also create opportunities to connect with other mothers. Engaging in conversations and sharing experiences during these classes can help forge meaningful connections.

Seek Online Communities: Explore online platforms and forums dedicated to postpartum recovery and motherhood. Online communities offer a space to connect with other mothers, exchange information, and seek support. Be mindful of choosing reliable and supportive communities that align with your values and needs.

Engage with Existing Networks: Reach out to family members, friends, and acquaintances who have gone through the postpartum experience. Joining existing networks of trusted individuals can provide a solid foundation of support during your recovery journey.

Chapter Twenty-Six

Postpartum Recovery Resources

The postpartum period is a transformative time in a woman's life, marked by physical and emotional changes as she recovers from childbirth and adjusts to life with a newborn. While this period can be both joyful and challenging, it is crucial for new mothers to have access to resources that can support their postpartum recovery. Below we will explore various postpartum recovery resources that can aid in physical healing, emotional well, being, and overall adjustment during this important phase.

Physical Recovery Resources:

Healthcare Providers: Your healthcare provider, such as an obstetrician or midwife, plays a vital role in your postpartum recovery. They can provide guidance, monitor your physical healing, and address any concerns or complications that may arise. Regular check, ups allow healthcare providers to assess your well, being and provide necessary interventions if needed.

Postpartum Care Packages: Many organizations and hospitals offer postpartum care packages, which include essential items for recovery, such as sanitary pads, nipple creams, perineal sprays, and herbal teas. These packages can be a valuable resource to ease discomfort and promote healing during the postpartum period.

Pelvic Floor Physiotherapy: Pelvic floor physiotherapy focuses on strengthening the pelvic floor muscles and addressing any pelvic floor issues that may arise postpartum, such as incontinence or pelvic organ prolapse. Working with a pelvic floor physiotherapist can help restore strength, function, and comfort in the pelvic area.

Lactation Consultants: Breastfeeding support is crucial for new mothers. Lactation consultants are trained professionals who can provide guidance, troubleshoot breastfeeding challenges, and offer tips to ensure successful breastfeeding. Their expertise can help enhance the breastfeeding experience and promote bonding with your baby.

Emotional Well, being Resources:

Postpartum Support Groups: Joining a postpartum support group allows you to connect with other new mothers who are experiencing similar challenges and emotions. These groups provide a safe space to share experiences, seek advice, and receive emotional support. They can help combat feelings of isolation and provide a sense of community during the postpartum period.

Mental Health Professionals: If you are experiencing postpartum depression, anxiety, or other mental health concerns, seeking help from a mental health professional is crucial. Therapists, counselors, and psychologists can provide individualized support and therapy to address your emotional well, being and mental health needs.

Online Communities and Forums: Online platforms and forums dedicated to postpartum recovery offer a wealth of information, resources, and support. They provide a space for connecting with other mothers, asking questions, and sharing experiences. However, it's important to engage with reputable and supportive communities to ensure accurate information and a positive online experience.

Self, care Practices: Engaging in self, care activities can significantly contribute to your emotional well, being during the postpartum period. Taking time for yourself, practicing mindfulness or meditation, engaging in hobbies, and prioritizing rest can help reduce stress, improve mood, and promote overall mental wellness.

Adjustment and Parenting Resources:

Parenting Classes and Workshops: Parenting classes offer valuable information and practical skills to navigate the challenges of newborn care, sleep routines, feeding techniques, and child development. These classes provide a supportive environment where you can learn from experienced educators and connect with other parents.

1Parenting Books and Blogs: There is a vast array of parenting books and blogs available that provide insight, guidance, and strategies for various parenting topics. These resources offer information on newborn care, sleep training, breastfeeding, and overall child development.

Books and Online Resources

The postpartum period is a transformative and challenging time for new mothers. It is a time of physical healing, emotional adjustment, and acquiring new parenting skills. In this modern age, there are numerous resources available to support women during their postpartum recovery. Books and online resources have become invaluable tools for providing information, guidance, and inspiration to navigate this unique journey. Below we will explore the importance of books and online resources in relation to postpartum recovery and discuss some notable recommendations.

Books for Postpartum Recovery:

Books have long been a trusted source of knowledge and inspiration. They offer in, depth information and personal stories that can empower and educate new mothers. Here are some noteworthy books on postpartum recovery:

"The Fourth Trimester: A Postpartum Guide to Healing Your Body, Balancing Your Emotions, and Restoring Your Vitality" by Kimberly Ann Johnson: This comprehensive guide addresses physical healing, emotional well, being, and spiritual growth during the postpartum period. It provides practical tips, self, care practices, and insights to navigate the challenges of the fourth trimester.

"The Postnatal Depletion Cure: A Complete Guide to Rebuilding Your Health and Reclaiming Your Energy for Mothers of Newborns, Toddlers, and Young Children" by Dr. Oscar Serrallach: This book focuses on the physical and emotional depletion that often accompanies early motherhood. It offers strategies to replenish vital nutrients, manage stress, and promote overall well, being.

"The First Forty Days: The Essential Art of Nourishing the New Mother" by Heng Ou: This book emphasizes the importance of rest, nourishment, and self, care during the initial forty days postpartum. It provides recipes, rituals, and guidance on nurturing the mother's physical and emotional well, being.

"Postnatal Pilates: A Recovery and Strength Exercise Program for New Moms" by Karrie Adamany: This book offers a safe and effective exercise program specifically designed for postpartum recovery. It focuses on rebuilding core strength, improving posture, and promoting overall fitness after childbirth.

Online Resources for Postpartum Recovery:

In addition to books, the digital age has opened up a vast array of online resources that provide accessible and up, to, date information on postpartum recovery. Here are some notable online resources for new mothers:

Websites and Blogs: Many reputable websites and blogs provide evidence, based information on postpartum recovery, including physical healing, breastfeeding support, emotional well, being, and parenting tips. Examples include BabyCenter, The Bump, and KellyMom.

Online Forums and Support Groups: Online forums and support groups offer a space for new mothers to connect, share experiences, and seek advice. These platforms allow for peer support and a sense of community during the postpartum journey. Examples include the Postpartum Support International forum and the What to Expect community.

Social Media: Social media platforms, such as Instagram and Facebook, have become valuable sources of information and inspiration for new mothers. Many experts and organizations share tips, resources, and personal stories related to postpartum recovery. Following reputable accounts and engaging in supportive communities can provide a sense of belonging and access to valuable resources.

Online Courses and Webinars: Various online courses and webinars cater specifically to postpartum recovery and parenting. These courses offer practical knowledge, strategies, and tools for navigating the postpartum period. Examples include courses on breastfeeding, baby care, self, care, and mental health.

Local Support Groups and Services

The postpartum period is a time of profound transformation for new mothers, both physically and emotionally. While it can be a joyful and fulfilling experience, it also comes with unique challenges and adjustments. Navigating this journey requires support, understanding, and connection with others who have shared similar experiences. Local support groups and services play a crucial role in providing this essential support network. Below we will explore the significance of local support groups and services in the context of postpartum recovery and highlight their benefits.

The Importance of Local Support Groups:

Local support groups offer a safe and nurturing environment where new mothers can connect with others facing similar challenges. These groups provide a space for sharing experiences, concerns, and triumphs. Here are some key reasons why local support groups are invaluable during the postpartum period:

a) Emotional Support: Adjusting to motherhood can be emotionally overwhelming. Local support groups provide an empathetic and non, judgmental space where women can express their feelings, validate their experiences, and receive support from others who understand firsthand the emotional ups and downs of the postpartum journey.

b) Shared Knowledge and Information: Local support groups offer a wealth of knowledge and information. Participants can learn from each other's experiences, gather practical tips, and gain insights into various aspects of postpartum recovery, such as breastfeeding, sleep issues, self, care, and infant care. This shared wisdom helps new mothers make informed decisions and feel more confident in their parenting choices.

c) Peer Bonding and Social Connection: Postpartum support groups foster a sense of belonging and camaraderie among participants. The shared experience of motherhood creates a unique bond, allowing women to forge lasting friendships and build a support network. This connection helps combat feelings of isolation and provides a valuable source of ongoing social support.

d) Normalizing Challenges: Postpartum support groups help normalize the challenges that new mothers may face. Hearing others' stories and struggles can alleviate feelings of inadequacy and reassure women that they are not alone in their experiences. It promotes a sense of solidarity and encourages self, compassion.

Types of Local Support Groups and Services:

Local communities offer various types of support groups and services tailored to meet the specific needs of postpartum women. Here are some examples of the support groups and services available:

a) Postpartum Support Groups: These groups focus on the emotional well, being of new mothers, addressing concerns such as postpartum depression, anxiety, and mood disorders. Facilitated by professionals or trained volunteers, these groups provide a safe space for sharing and seeking guidance on managing emotional challenges.

b) Breastfeeding Support Groups: Breastfeeding can be a significant aspect of postpartum recovery. Breastfeeding support groups offer guidance, troubleshooting, and encouragement to women who may encounter difficulties in breastfeeding. These groups provide expert advice from lactation consultants and the opportunity to connect with other breastfeeding mothers.

c) Parenting Classes: Local communities often organize parenting classes that cover a range of topics, including newborn care, infant feeding, sleep strategies, and postpartum self, care. These classes allow new parents to learn valuable skills, ask questions, and gain confidence in their caregiving abilities.

d) Exercise and Wellness Programs: Physical activity is essential for postpartum recovery. Local fitness centers or community organizations may offer specialized exercise classes tailored to the needs of postpartum women. These classes focus on rebuilding strength, improving posture, and promoting overall well, being.

e) Doula Services: Doulas provide emotional and practical support during pregnancy, birth, and the postpartum period. They offer non, medical assistance, such as helping with breastfeeding, providing household support, and offering guidance on newborn care.

Chapter Twenty-Seven

Celebrating Your Journey

Bringing a new life into the world is a transformative experience for women. The postpartum period, often referred to as the fourth trimester, is a time of physical healing and emotional adjustment. It is a remarkable journey that deserves to be celebrated. Below we will explore the significance of celebrating the postpartum recovery journey and its impact on women's well, being. From acknowledging achievements to embracing self, care, Below we will delve into various aspects of celebration during the postpartum period.

Recognizing Milestones and Achievements:

The postpartum recovery journey is filled with milestones and achievements, both big and small. It is essential for women to acknowledge and celebrate these milestones as they mark significant progress in their recovery. Here are some examples:

a) Physical Recovery: From healing incisions to regaining strength and mobility, every step towards physical recovery is worth celebrating. It could be as simple as being able to walk a little farther each day or having a pain, free day.

b) Emotional Well, being: The emotional roller coaster of the postpartum period can be challenging. Celebrating moments of emotional stability, practicing self, compassion, and seeking support when needed are important achievements.

c) Nurturing the Baby: Each milestone reached by the baby, such as the first smile or sleeping through the night, is a testament to the mother's love and care. Celebrating these moments strengthens the bond between mother and child.

d) Self, Care: Taking care of oneself is crucial during the postpartum recovery period. Celebrating small acts of self, care, such as enjoying a hot bath or indulging in a hobby, reinforces the importance of prioritizing one's well, being.

Embracing Support and Community:

Celebrating the postpartum recovery journey is not a solitary endeavor. It is essential to embrace the support of loved ones and the wider community. Here are some ways to foster a sense of celebration through support and community:

a) Partner Support: Recognizing and appreciating the role of a partner in the postpartum recovery journey is vital. Partners can provide emotional support, assist with childcare, and celebrate milestones together. Expressing gratitude and acknowledging their contributions can strengthen the bond between partners.

b) Family and Friends: Surrounding oneself with a supportive network of family and friends is invaluable during the postpartum period. They can offer assistance, lend a listening ear, and share in the joy of milestones achieved. Celebrating with loved ones can foster a sense of connection and belonging.

c) Online Communities: The digital age has opened doors to virtual communities where women can connect with others going through similar experiences. Online forums, social media groups, and support networks provide opportunities for sharing stories, seeking advice, and celebrating achievements together.

d) Support Groups: Joining postpartum support groups can provide a sense of camaraderie and validation. These groups offer a platform to share experiences, receive guidance, and celebrate milestones collectively. Interacting with other women who are on a similar journey can be empowering and uplifting.

Practicing Self, Care and Well, being:

Self, care is an integral part of postpartum recovery and should be celebrated as an act of self, love and nourishment. Here are some aspects of self, care that deserve recognition:

a) Rest and Sleep: Celebrating moments of rest and quality sleep is essential for physical and emotional well, being. Napping when the baby naps, prioritizing sleep hygiene, and seeking help to ensure adequate rest are important steps towards recovery.

Acknowledging Your Strength

The postpartum period is a time of immense change, both physically and emotionally, for women who have recently given birth. It is a transformative journey that requires strength and resilience. Below we will explore the importance of acknowledging and celebrating the strength of women during the postpartum recovery process. From the physical challenges of childbirth to the emotional adjustments of motherhood, we will discuss the various aspects that demonstrate the remarkable strength of women during this period.

Physical Strength:

Childbirth is a physically demanding experience, and the body goes through significant changes during and after delivery. Acknowledging and appreciating the physical strength that women exhibit during this time is crucial. Here are some aspects to consider:

a) Labor and Delivery: The process of labor and delivery requires tremendous physical endurance. Women endure hours of contractions and exertion, showcasing their resilience and strength.

b) Recovery from Birth: Following childbirth, the body undergoes a healing process. Acknowledging the body's ability to heal and regenerate is essential. From healing incisions to recovering strength and mobility, women demonstrate remarkable resilience.

c) Caring for the Baby: The physical demands of caring for a newborn, such as lifting, feeding, and soothing, require strength and stamina. Women adapt to these new responsibilities and develop physical endurance as they care for their little ones.

Emotional Strength:

The postpartum period is not only physically demanding but also emotionally challenging. Women experience a range of emotions as they navigate the joys and complexities of motherhood. Recognizing and celebrating their emotional strength is equally important. Consider the following:

a) Hormonal Changes: The fluctuation of hormones during the postpartum period can lead to mood swings and emotional vulnerability. Coping with these changes and maintaining emotional well, being requires immense strength.

b) Sleep Deprivation: Lack of sleep can significantly impact a person's emotional state. Managing sleep deprivation while attending to the needs of a newborn requires resilience and emotional strength.

c) Adjusting to Motherhood: Becoming a mother is a life, altering experience. Women must adapt to new roles, responsibilities, and challenges. Navigating this transition with patience, love, and self, compassion demonstrates incredible emotional strength.

Self, Care and Well, being:

Acknowledging one's strength also involves recognizing the importance of self, care and well, being during the postpartum period. Here are some areas to consider:

a) Prioritizing Self, Care: Taking care of oneself is vital for physical and emotional recovery. This includes practices such as rest, proper nutrition, engaging in activities that bring joy, and seeking support when needed. Recognizing the value of self, care and taking steps to prioritize it demonstrate strength and self, awareness.

b) Seeking Support: Recognizing the need for support and actively seeking it is a sign of strength. Whether it's reaching out to friends and family, joining support groups, or seeking professional help, asking for support demonstrates courage and resilience.

c) Mental Health: Postpartum mental health is a significant aspect of recovery. Acknowledging and addressing mental health challenges, such as postpartum depression or anxiety, requires strength and self, awareness. Seeking professional help and engaging in therapeutic practices contribute to overall well, being.

Empowering Others:

Acknowledging one's strength can also inspire and empower other women. By openly sharing their experiences, challenges, and triumphs, women can create a supportive community and uplift others who may be going through similar journeys. Celebrating each other's strength and accomplishments fosters a sense of solidarity and empowerment.

Embracing Your New Normal

The journey of postpartum recovery is a unique and transformative experience for new mothers. It is a time of physical healing, emotional adjustments, and adapting to the responsibilities of caring for a newborn. Below we will explore the concept of embracing your new normal during the postpartum period. We will discuss the various aspects of postpartum recovery and how women can navigate this phase while embracing the changes and challenges that come with it.

Physical Recovery:

The physical recovery after childbirth is a significant part of the postpartum period. It involves healing from the strains of pregnancy and delivery. Embracing your new normal in terms of physical changes can be empowering. Consider the following:

a) Body Image: Pregnancy and childbirth bring about changes in a woman's body. Embracing these changes and accepting the postpartum body is essential for self, acceptance and self, love. Recognizing that the body has accomplished a remarkable feat and allowing it to heal and regain strength is a part of embracing your new normal.

b) Rest and Self, Care: Postpartum recovery requires adequate rest and self, care. Embracing your new normal means prioritizing self, care, listening to your body's needs, and giving yourself the time and space to recover physically. This may involve getting enough sleep, eating nourishing meals, and engaging in gentle exercises as advised by healthcare professionals.

c) Physical Activities: As the body heals, gradually incorporating physical activities can be a part of embracing your new normal. Consultation with healthcare professionals is crucial to determine when and how to safely engage in exercises and activities that support your physical recovery. Embracing your new normal also means finding a balance between rest and gradually increasing your physical activity levels.

Emotional Adjustment:

Embracing your new normal after childbirth involves acknowledging and navigating the emotional changes that come with becoming a mother. The postpartum period can bring about a range of emotions, and understanding and accepting these feelings is crucial. Consider the following:

a) Postpartum Hormonal Changes: Hormonal shifts after childbirth can contribute to mood swings, baby blues, or postpartum depression. Embracing your new normal means recognizing and seeking support if needed. Communicating openly with loved ones and healthcare professionals about your emotional well, being can help in navigating these changes.

b) Bonding with Your Baby: Building a strong bond with your baby is a significant part of embracing your new normal. It takes time to establish this connection, and every mother, baby relationship is unique. Embrace the process of getting to know your baby, understanding their cues, and fostering a loving and nurturing environment.

c) Mental Health Support: Prioritizing mental health is an important aspect of postpartum recovery. Embracing your new normal means seeking professional help if you experience symptoms of postpartum depression, anxiety, or other mental health challenges. It is not a sign of weakness but rather a step toward self, care and overall well, being.

Building a Support System:

Embracing your new normal can be made easier with a strong support system. Surrounding yourself with supportive individuals who understand and empathize with the challenges of postpartum recovery is essential. Consider the following:

a) Partner Support: Building a strong support system begins with the support of your partner. Communicate openly with your partner about your needs and expectations during the postpartum period. Embracing your new normal together as a couple can strengthen your bond and make the journey smoother.

SD - #0142 - 070926 - C0 - 229/152/13 - PB - 9781776847068 - Matt Lamination